M. Allegretti

The Therapeutic Properties of Electromagnetic Waves

From Pulsed Fields to Rifing

Copyright © 2018 Ing. Marcello Allegretti

All rights reserved.

ISBN: 9781719822237
ISBN-13:

ACKNOWLEDGMENTS

There are many events, stimuli and friends, which have led me to write this book.

Therefore, I wish to thank the following people:

My friend Natale Petti, Director of the Aron Schools (Bari, Italy), for his teachings, his support, his suggestions and his generosity,

John White, a great scientist, who is revolutionizing the world of Rifing and a friend who intrigued me and compelled me to conquer the world of frequencies and my research",

Leonardo Righini, who, with his experience and technical preparation, has helped me dissolve doubts and provided information and helpful ideas in electrotherapy and magnetotherapy,

Domenico Cantatore, for his invaluable contribution in the scientific revision of the text,

Stefano Marcuzzo, for his contribution in the notions of neuroacoustics,

Irene Gomulka, for her experience and for the revision of the English text,

All those who supported me and encouraged me in my studies and research,

All the Friends, who with their suggestions and indications, helped me make this book better,

And finally… my son Marco, who inspires and stimulates me every day in my studies and research.

Legal Notice & Disclaimer

This book is a work to be considered as a notional aid for the knowledge of techniques and application methods of electronic devices, which use electromagnetic fields for various purposes. The information contained herein is not intended as, and should not be used for, therapeutic, diagnostic or prescriptive purposes, nor to prevent, treat or cure disease, but for education and responsible experimentation only.

The information this book contains can in no way replace the work of a medically trained professional. Please consult a licensed health practitioner for medical advice.

The author cannot guarantee the reliability of the information contained herein and there are no errors and/or omissions. The information and concepts within this guide must not be considered or construed in any way to be medical advice or treatment.

The author of this book cannot be held liable for any consequences, harmful or otherwise, that may occur by using the information contained in this book.

CONTENTS

Preface	7
Preface by John White	9
Introduction	11
The reactions of cells and tissues exposed to electromagnetic fields	13
- The electrical properties of cells and organic tissues	20
- Measurements that can be performed on a human body	24
Electroacupuncture according to Voll (EAV)	25
Bioelectrical Impedance Analysis	27
Non-linear Diagnostic Systems (NLS)	32
- Effects of electro-magnetic fields	35
Effects of electromagnetic waves at low frequencies	35
Effects of electromagnetic waves at high frequencies	37
The harmful effects of electromagnetic waves	39
Application technologies for electromagnetic waves	43
- Therapies with light radiation	43
- Electrostatic therapy	48
- Electrotherapy or Electrostimulation	49
Micro Current Electrical Stimulation (MET)	50
Neuromuscular Electrical Stimulation Devices (NMES)	52
Functional Electrical Stimulation (FES)	53
Transcutaneous Electrical Nerve Stimulation (TENS)	54
Cranial electrotherapy stimulation (CES)	54
H-wave	55
Percutaneous Electrical Nerve Stimulation (PENS)	55
Percutaneous Neuromodulation Therapy (PNT)	55
High Voltage Galvanic Stimulation (HVGS)	55
Electroacupuncture (EAP)	56
Electrostimulation of acupuncture points	58
- Thermotherapy	59
Infrared rays	60
Radar or Microwave therapy	61
Marconitherapy	62
Tecar-Therapy	62

Hyperthermia in oncology	64
- Ultrasound therapy	66
- Extracorporeal Shockwave Therapy (ESWT)	67
- Neuroacoustics	69
- Magnetotherapy	72
Repetitive Transcranial Magnetic Stimulation (rTMS)	73
High-frequency magnetotherapy	73
Low-frequency magnetic therapy	74
PEMF (Pulsed Electro-Magnetic Fields)	74
- Rifing	76

Pulsed Electro-Magnetic Fields (PEMF) 77
- Effects on cells 78
- Therapeutic applications 80
- Pain 82
- The regeneration of tissues.. 83
    Musculoskeletal disorders... 83
    Bone healing.. 84
    Nervous tissues 86
- Conclusions on PEMF 88

NASA's research on electromagnetic waves 89

Rifing... 97
- Dr. Royal Raymond Rife 97
- How Rifing works... 103
- Healing 104
- Detox 109
- Killing 110
- The Herxheimer reaction 119
- The frequencies of Rifing 121
- Waveforms 124
- When the frequencies do not work 132
- The methods of application 133

Considerations on the technologies examined 143
- The emission power... 144
- Biological and therapeutic effects... 145
- Final reflections 151

Preface

Everything is information; this is the assumption of quantum physics. Professor Carlo Rubbia, an internationally renowned scientist, won the Nobel Prize with a formula that shows that we are able to observe only one billionth of the characteristics of an object.

Current physics tells us that we know at most five percent of the reality that surrounds us, the rest is made of dark matter, that is invisible to our eyes and to the tools we have available to measure it and therefore unknown to us. The present medical science seems to have detached itself from the laws of physics and nature, denying the evident existence of the laws that regulate the basic functions of our body. Just talking about quantum physics and quantum medicine to our doctors is uncomfortable! However, the truth is that they cannot define their scientific discipline without accepting science in its entirety.

The human body consists of apparatuses, which are made up of organs, made of tissues, composed of cells, in turn made up of organelles, composed of macromolecules, constructed from molecules, and at the base of all these, we have atoms. At the root of the human Biology, is Physics, because at the base of the human body there are the atoms.

Physics is the only true science, which exists as the only discipline that can be confirmed through the scientific method. To deny the effects of physics, which considers the atom as a basic unit on human health, is like not accepting that a house made of bricks, which is composed of earth or clay. We accept that the quality of the bricks as fundamental, but we do not consider that the clay that composes them is fundamental and some even deny the influence of the clay itself. It is absurd to believe that some are able to think that!

A curious and ethical scientist, faced with empirical and repeatable evidence that he cannot explain, wonders what he has not understood or what function unknown to him can allow this phenomenon. He does not say that the phenomenon is not true, only because he cannot explain it. This is not scientific and leaves no room for growth to our science.

The body is a holistic system that must be analyzed, viewed and considered at many levels: Biological, Psychological and Informational, therefore Quantum, specifying that the quantum reading does not exclude the relative Einsteinian one. I mean that the laws of quantum physics and those of relative physics collaborate in giving us the most complete reading we could ever have to date.

It is obvious and proven that nutrition is a fundamental component for human health. Food can change the fate of our tissues and our cells, as it could also change, if we were exposed to radiation, chemicals, toxic substances, emotional stresses and traumas, substances or microorganisms. After what has been affirmed, it seems quite obvious that we must take care of our body.

The frequency, electromagnetic, informational and scalar approaches, allow the body to be treated in a non-invasive way and, if well used, can give truly impressive results. Of course, with applying the investigative systems and the various treatments, you will begin to experience a healthy change, which must be integrated with various other methods, as needed. This is the vision I have been proposing for years with the BioPsicoQuantistica, an integrated system that recognizes the various and very different skills according to need, a system which, by rejecting every fundamentalist approach, recognizes a probable aid in every discipline or instrument of treatment. In this vision, the use of electromagnetic waves is a valuable evaluation and treatment tool, in an integrated and holistic perspective.

I am, therefore, very happy to be able to comment on this work done by my dear and esteemed friend Marcello Allegretti, a trained scientist, a man of great heart, culture and humility. For about 20 years, Marcello has been involved in search of informational therapies. He has been able to describe very complicated topics in a concise and simple way, in which to make them understandable even to non-professionals. Nothing could be more natural for someone like him, who in his previous publications had me amazed at the completeness and precision of his works, which always appear to be meticulous and at the same time simple to comprehend. After reading this text, there was a sentence that came out of my mouth quite spontaneously and I exclaimed: "Finally a book in which someone spoke in a precise, simple, concise and scientific way about informational therapies!" This is a very useful book, which is necessary for operators in this sector and especially for those who are doing Treatments or Quantum Therapies, as if they were the latest discovery of modern magic. This book, which speaks of Science, will be able to teach many.

To the readers of this book, remember, that in terms of health, the multifactorial always applies to different levels and that utilizing only one approach always proves to be poor and limited. To the skeptics, I say that curiosity is at the base of the impulse, which has driven every scientist. So give it a try and maybe you can change your mind.

Dr. Natale Petti
Clinical Psychologist and Naturopath BPQ

Preface

by John White

In 1931, the world celebrated "The End of All Disease." The answer to illnesses had been found; electromagnetic waves. Independent clinical trials confirmed that cancer had been conquered. Then the unbelievable happened.

Faced with a disastrous loss of drug income, authorities decided to censor the information. The genius who had discovered the answer to disease eventually died a broken man.

Large corporation decisions made are based on earnings, market share and growth. Ethics and morals play second-fiddle to profit. The casualty in the drive for prosperity is humanity. Yet, true wealth is health.

My name is John White. I created the Spooky2 health system, write the Spooky2 software and develop the Spooky2 hardware. My goal is to empower people with knowledge and equipment, so they can take control over their own health.

Marcello and I are close friends. We first exchanged emails in 2016, when he kindly offered to translate the Spooky2 manual into Italian; his mother tongue. Since then, we have kept in contact to exchange ideas. Nevertheless, it came as a surprise when Marcello asked me to write a preface for his new book.

I was fortunate to meet Marcello in person during the Italian portion of the 2017 Spooky2 European tour. What struck me most about him was his astonishing enthusiasm and energy. His strive for perfection and eye for detail is only surpassed by his love of his family, for he is blessed with a loving wife and two wonderful sons.

Marcello Allegretti is an exceptional electronics and medical expert who has an innate ability to transform complex concepts in a language we can all understand. What others struggle with, Marcello takes in his stride. As you read each chapter, you will understand concepts which even experts may find difficult to comprehend. This is the Marcello magic.

In a previous book titled: *The frequencies of Rifing*, Marcello listed the frequencies, which are best suited for different health conditions. In this book, Marcello goes further, and explains how frequencies actually work.

Marcello begins by describing how electromagnetic fields affect body tissue, and why frequency is so important. Each frequency can affect the body in different ways.

The next chapter reveals the many ways electromagnetic fields can be applied. Never shy of detail, Marcello covers the full spectrum, from light waves down to temperature.

Pulsed magnetic fields can markedly reduce recovery time. NASA used these fields for astronauts during missions. A self-treatment method was developed using PEMF (Pulsed Electromagnetic Field) devices. Marcello dedicates an entire chapter to this important subject.

The final chapters discuss Rifing. A term, which means applying precise frequencies to resonate and destroy pathogens. At the beginning of this preface, I talked about the "The End of All Disease," which was celebrated back in 1931. A man had discovered the cure for cancer, tuberculosis, tetanus and much more. His name was Royal Raymond Rife. The terms *"Rife" treatments* and *"Rifing"* are in memory of this great man.

Imagine a world without disease. Royal Rife found the answer over 80 years ago. *The Therapeutic Properties of Electromagnetic Waves* ensures this solution is not forgotten.

So read on, intrepid reader. Electromagnetic waves can indeed heal. And, you are about to discover how!

John White

Introduction

The growing interest and use of technologies that utilize electromagnetic waves for therapeutic purposes and the exponential increase of scientific publications on this subject, have pushed me to try to gather all the information possible, in order to clarify first of all to me, which methods can be used to achieve the most benefits and with the quickest solutions, as this is necessary when you are afflicted by a health problem.

Embracing and explaining, at least in a summary way, such a wide range of applications with electromagnetic waves has not been easy, since the technologies used are from the beginning of the last century to date, and are many. These notions are therefore addressed to a very large audience, which includes researchers, doctors, holistic operators, electronic technicians or specialists in bioengineering, but also any person who has an interest in deepening or learning more about these topics and can then decide if and how to use them in the most targeted way. For this reason I have tried to use a language that everyone can understand and maybe I have elaborated on explanations that for some may seem completely superfluous or trivial.

Another of the fundamental purposes of this book is to try to offer all the most reliable scientific explanations concerning the mechanisms of interaction between electromagnetic fields and organic tissues. It is absolutely normal for every researcher to try to demonstrate and illustrate how a series of electrical, chemical and biological reactions can take place and then produce certain results. Many have given plausible and satisfying explanations; several others have come to identical conclusions. All the articles that I had the opportunity to review have focused on describing the biological effects (e.g., increase in cell membrane potential), and almost never understanding or pointing out that the real effect of the electromagnetic waves, is that the electromagnetic waves lead to stimulation genetics.

Fortunately, this goal has been achieved by NASA, which, thanks to the in-depth studies, carried out in its well-equipped laboratories, has finally provided a precise and detailed scientific explanation. Probably only NASA could do it, since independent researchers do not have the necessary resources and pharmaceutical companies have no interest in such technologies, which often oppose or discredit such research.

Finally, when all the possible interpretations offered by the scientific world are still not enough, it remains only *something* immaterial, which cannot be explained satisfactorily with traditional theories: it is the content of *information* that an electromagnetic signal can provide. In this case, only quantum physics can help us. Understanding a phenomenon that can be explained with such theories can be quite complicated, so, we can all at least verify its practical effects, the empirical results. These topics will be dealt with in the second to the last chapter of this book.

Lastly, I think it is important to point out that some of the topics discussed, in particular those concerning Rifing and pathogens, can be considered by most of the scientific community as having no solid foundation and clinical trials to prove its effectiveness. Many of the theories encountered, have been and still are opposed by the medical and scientific community, despite the surprising results obtained. However, since these technologies are officially used in many countries, I thought it useful to provide all the latest concepts for your review. It will take some time and evolution to establish its truthfulness and effectiveness.

> *Each doctrine passes through three phases:*
> *It is attacked and declared absurd.*
> *Then it is admitted that it is true and evident, but irrelevant.*
> *In the end, its real importance is recognized*
> *and his detractors claim the honor of having discovered it.*
>
> **William Jones**

The reactions of cells and tissues exposed to electromagnetic fields

Many people are currently thinking that a satisfactory explanation for using electromagnetic fields on the cells of living organisms with different frequencies and waveforms is still lacking. This depends first of all on the incomplete knowledge of the phenomena at the genetic level, of the cellular membrane, of the organelles contained within it, of the extracellular matrix and in general of the structural complexity of the biological tissues and their inhomogeneity. Nevertheless, we will try to expose the most accredited hypotheses, which the research carried out in this sector offers us.

To understand how normal and then pulsed electromagnetic waves can act on an organism and in particular on cells and tissues, it is first necessary to recall some simple concepts of physics.

Sinusoidal Wave: the entire waveform has the great importance. It is actually a very simple and natural curve, which underlies many physical phenomena.

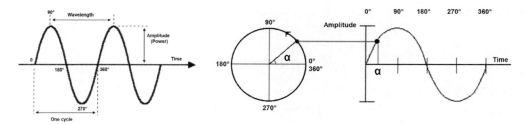

The sound is made of sinusoidal waves and so are the light, the voltage and the electric current supply to our homes. Sinusoids are the fundamental "bricks" with which any other waveform can be constructed. In practice, by adding different sine waves with different frequencies and amplitudes, any signal can be created with any waveform.

Wavelength: it is the distance in meters of a complete oscillation, or the distance between two maximum points (crests) or two minima (valleys) of an electromagnetic wave. It is represented with the Greek letter λ and is linked to the frequency through the relation λ = c / f where: λ is the wavelength expressed in meters; **c** is the speed of light expressed in meters per second. From this expression, it is inferred that the higher the frequency, the shorter the wavelength.

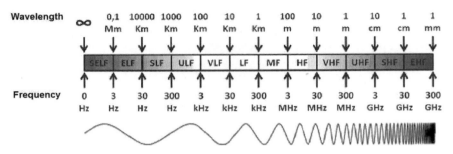

Frequency: it is the number of cycles or oscillations of a waveform per second; the unit of measure is the hertz (Hz). Frequency is the parameter that influences more than any other, the mode of interaction of an electromagnetic field with a biological system. For example, the depth of penetration of electromagnetic waves in the tissues of the human body is inversely proportional to the frequency: in practice, when the frequencies are lower, then they can go deeper. Frequencies up to 30 MHz can penetrate all the tissues of the human body, up to the bones. The very high frequencies used, for example, the mobile telephones (some GHz), have a penetration power of about 1-2 cm. Furthermore, various other electrical parameters, such as the permittivity and conductivity of biological tissues; vary according to the frequency applied.

Harmonics: in physics, they are frequencies whose value is an integer multiple of the fundamental frequency of a wave. For example, if the fundamental frequency is 1 kHz, its second harmonic is 1 kHz x 2 = 2 kHz, the third 3 kHz, the fourth 4 kHz and so on. Similarly, a sub-harmonic is a whole submultiple of

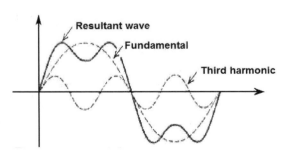

the fundamental frequency, so the second sub-harmonic of 1 kHz is 1 kHz / 2 = 500 Hz, the third sub-harmonic 1 kHz / 3, etc. Frequently, instead of using this criterion, it is preferred to use as a multiplier or divisor, the octave (as in music); in this case every octave is twice the previous one (e.g., 1kHz, 2 kHz, 4kHz, 8 kHz, etc.) Similarly, the lower octaves are half of the previous ones. By comparing the two multipliers, we can easily identify the mathematical relationship between harmonics and octaves: for example the third octave higher than 1 kHz, i.e., 8 kHz, corresponds to the 8th harmonic. Therefore, the octaves could be defined as "special" harmonics.

Amplitude: it is the height of a crest or a half-wave; it can correspond to a voltage (V), a current (A) or other electrical or magnetic parameters.

Voltage: is the difference between the electrical potential of two points, such as the poles of a battery or those of an electrical outlet. In these cases, the difference is that the voltage of a battery is continuous or has a constant value over time (graphically a straight line parallel to the abscissa axis); the voltage of an electrical outlet (like the domestic ones) is alternated, that is, variable over time at the frequency of 50/60 Hz, with a sinusoidal trend and therefore with the poles that are inverted (from positive to negative) 50/60 times a second. The voltage is measured in volts (V).

Current: it is a displacement of electric charges, a flow of electrons from a negative to a positive pole. When this movement travels through a conductive material (like a copper wire), we can imagine it as a stream of water flowing through a pipe. As for the voltage, the current can be continuous or alternating over time. The current is measured in ampere (A).

Intensity: it is the quantity of energy that flows and is proportional to the square of the amplitude (it is measured in W / m2). Each electromagnetic wave is characterized by a power and a transport of energy, which results to be proportional to the product of the intensities of the electric field and of the magnetic field. It is important to know that the power decreases with the square of the distance from the source: for example, at a double distance one quarter of the power is collected.

Electric Field: it is a field of forces generated in space by the presence of electric charges. This field is always created by an electric voltage and is directly proportional to its amplitude (so the higher the voltage, the stronger the resulting electric field will be); it is represented with the symbol "E" and is measured in volts per meter (V / m). It manifests itself in any electrical component under voltage and, unlike the magnetic one; it is emitted even when no current flows.

The electric fields act in depth, in all the tissues and in all the bodily regions and they fall as a function of the square of the distance.

If the field strength is almost *equal* to that of the cell potential, the electric field promotes an ionic current of endocellular capacitive displacement (that resides inside the cell) that propagates inside the cells, following the flow lines of the exogenous field.

If the exogenous potential (created by the external electric field) is *greater* than the endocellular one, the cell faces the exogenous charges with equal endogenous charges, but with opposite sign, preventing the exogenous potential to disturb the endocellular electrochemical balance.

Magnetic field: it is the force field produced by a magnet, or by an electric current, or by a variable electric field over time. It is represented with the symbol H and is measured in amperes per meter (A / m), in tesla (more commonly in µT - micro tesla) or in gauss (1 gauss = 0.0001 tesla). The alternating magnetic field is therefore directly proportional to the current value and occurs when the latter runs through an electrical conductor; the field becomes very powerful when the conductors are arranged in turns.

Actions of the magnetic fields are associated with their spatial distribution; the magnetic field decays proportionally to the inverse of the distance cube. For example, a magnetic field that has an intensity of 1000 gauss at one meter, at a distance of 3 meters from the source, the intensity will be reduced to 12.3 gauss (= 1 / 3^3x1000, which corresponds to a reduction of 81 times).

To have parameters of comparison with the values that will be subsequently declared, it is useful to know that:
- The earth's magnetic field varies from about 70 µT to the poles, to 25 µT at the equator with an average of 50 µT at other latitudes;
- A large magnet could have a field of 10 gauss (0,001 T);
- A magnetic resonance machine can generate fields up to 7 tesla.

Electromagnetic field: it is the combination of the electric field and the magnetic field and it propagates in the form of electromagnetic waves. Depending on the source of emission of these fields, there is not always the simultaneous presence of both. For example, near a radiating source, the electric field and the magnetic field can be considered separately (this occurs above all, at very low frequencies); for distances greater than about one tenth of the wavelength, the two fields concatenate and propagate in the free space in the form of an electromagnetic field.

As the frequency increases, the energy carried by an electromagnetic wave increases proportionally.

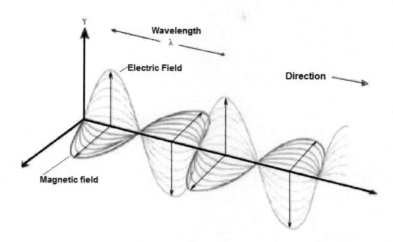

An **electric field** also *exists* when there is *no current flowing* (just the presence of a voltage). In contrast, a **magnetic field** *does not exist if there is no current circulation.*

Furthermore, electric and magnetic fields are not mutually exclusive. For example, charged particles when they move generate magnetic fields; similarly, if the magnetic field changes over time, it will generate electric fields.

Scalar Fields: were discovered by James Clark Maxwell, a Scottish scientist born in 1831, who formulated theories on electromagnetic radiation and electromagnetic fields. Nikola Tesla discovered this new form of energy in the late 1800s, while performing experiments with powerful and fast DC electric discharges. Later Tesla, managed to use them to transport electricity from a transmitting station to a receiver, even at great distances, without loss of energy and without the need for cables. With this technology, not only was the transmission of energy possible, but also the almost instantaneous and precise wireless transmission of any type of information, signals, messages or characters, to all parts of the world. In the 21st century, they were called **scalar waves**.

As for electromagnetic (transverse) waves, as shown above, the fields oscillate in orthogonal directions with respect to the propagation, those scalars oscillate in the direction of propagation (longitudinal), as in the case of mechanical or sound waves that move only along the propagation direction.

Electromagnetic waves, in addition to the transverse component, also have a longitudinal component that is small at low frequencies, but becomes prevalent at higher frequencies. When the frequencies become extremely high, the transverse component becomes negligible, while the longitudinal component becomes predominant.

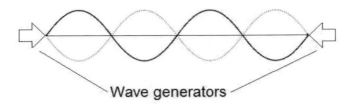

The scalar wave is the wave that remains when two opposing electromagnetic fields interfere, canceling, as in Tesla's experiments, the electrical and magnetic components (it can be created by two opposed electromagnetic waves, 180° out of phase temporally). The result is a longitudinal wave, which vibrates in the same direction in which it travels.

Different researchers believe that scalar fields can be described as *torsion fields, Zero-point Energy (ZPE), non-hertzian waves, orgone*, or in areas other than physics, such as subtle energies: *ether, etheric, world spiritual, Qi or prana*.

According to Dr. Konstantin Meyl, Professor of Electronics, scalar waves can be transferred to human DNA, since our DNA is a quantum antenna capable of receiving and transmitting magnetic scalar waves. About twenty years ago, Prof. Meyl discovered and proved the existence of both electric and magnetic scalar waves. Tesla discovered the electric scalar wave, and proved its existence. The magnetic scalar wave is the one with greater biological relevance, since most communication between cells is done using this wave type.

Resonance: it is a phenomenon that is obtained when an oscillating system is subjected to a periodic force of frequency equal to the system's own frequency. Generally, it causes a significant increase in the amplitude of the oscillations and therefore a considerable accumulation of energy within the stressed system, which can eventually destroy the system.

Conductivity: it is the ability of a material to conduct an electric current (it is the inverse of **Resistivity**); in organic tissues it can be influenced by:
- Temperature variations,
- Oxygen levels,

- Concentrations of intracellular minerals and extracellular fluids,
- Types of intracellular minerals present and extracellular fluids,
- pH (both intracellular and extracellular),
- Level of hydration (water contained outside and inside the cells),
- Relationship between structured/unstructured water inside the cell,
- Lipid membrane/sterol,
- Free radical activity,
- Amount of negative charges present on the surface of cell membranes,
- Quantity and structure of hyaluronic acid in the extracellular matrix,
- Endogenous electric fields,
- External application of electromagnetic fields,
- Presence of electrophilic chemical toxins and heavy metals both within the cell in the extracellular matrix.

All the parameters described above are linked to each other and each influences the effects they can have on an extremely complex and delicate system such as the biological one: frequency, waveform, intensity, resonance, polarization and modulation play a role of fundamental importance, as we will illustrate later.

The electrical properties of cells and organic tissues

The body is a complex electrical machine and the cells and tissues that make up the human body possess different electrical properties. The energetic communication of the body does not take place exclusively through the nervous system. Among the electrical properties that cells manifest, there is the ability to conduct electrical energy, to generate it and to create electromagnetic fields.

Biological tissues cannot only receive, transduce and transmit electrical signals, but also acoustic, magnetic, mechanical, thermal vibrations and photons signal. This is why it is possible to see phenomena such as:
- Biological reactions to the geomagnetic fields of the earth and to the Schumann fields,
- Biological reactions to the atmospheric electromagnetic field and disturbances due to sunspots, thunder, lightning and earthquakes,
- Biological responses to heat and light,
- Biological responses to frequency generators that produce waves and electric fields, magnetic, photons, acoustic vibrations,
- Biological reactions under the hands of a pranotherapist.

In biological organisms, the negatively charged carriers are the electrons or ions that have acquired an electron, while the ions that have lost an electron are positively charged. For example, sodium ions, potassium, calcium, magnesium have a positive charge, while those of chlorine have a negative charge.

The **cell**, the basic element of living organisms, is characterized by a membrane that separates it from the surrounding environment (extracellular matrix), making it an entity capable of interacting with the external environment.

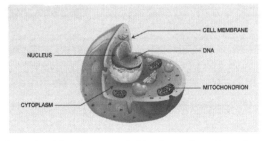

Cell membranes are composed of a double layer of lipid molecules that electrically behave like an insulator (dielectric). This property has the function of limiting the movement of charged ions and electrons, which can in any case cross the membrane by means of specialized ion channels.

The cell membrane is permeable to ions (in particular to sodium and potassium) in a selective manner, therefore different concentrations of these and other mineral ions are created on both sides of the membrane, which lead to an imbalance of the electric charges between the inside of the cell and the outside. The difference in electrical potential, measurable between the liquid inside a cell (cytosol), which has negative charges and the extracellular space, which has positive charges, is called **Membrane Potential**. All healthy living cells have a membrane potential between **-60** and **-100mV**. The membrane potential creates an electrochemical force that regulates the chemical exchange (permeability), through the cell for the control of nutrients, proteins, enzymes, etc.

Healthy cells maintain a high concentration of potassium ions and a low concentration of sodium ions inside, but when the cells are sick, sodium and water flows inside, while potassium, magnesium, calcium and zinc are reduced within the cell, decreasing the membrane potential up to values that can reach **-20mV**.

The potential difference on the two sides of the cell membrane creates a strong electric field that represents an available source of energy for a significant number of cellular activities including membrane transport and the generation of electrical impulses in the brain, nerves, heart and muscles. This electric field is surprisingly high: 10,000,000 Volts / m according to Reilly[1] and up to 20 million Volts / m according to Brown[2]. A very high potential is also created on the membranes of the mitochondria. Positively charged hydrogen ions are maintained in a high concentration outside the mitochondrial membrane by the action of the electron transport chain, which creates a mitochondrial membrane potential of about 40,000,000 volts / m.

Dr. Merrill Garnett[3] has long studied the role of charge displacements and the flow of electric current in the cell (biocurrents). He believes that biological molecules of liquid crystals and structures such as hyaluronic acid, prothrombin, DNA, cytoskeletal proteins and cell membranes, are involved in the maintenance of a current both inwards and outwards of the cell. The current inward flows from the cell membrane to the cellular structures such as the mitochondria and the DNA and is involved in the activation of the DNA and in the creation of an electric field

---

[1] Reilly JP. *Applied Bioelectricity: From Electrical Stimulation to Electropathology.* New York: Springer, 1998.

[2] Brown G. *The Energy of Life: The Science of What Makes Our Minds and Bodies Work.* New York, NY: The Free Press, 1999

[3] Garnett M. *First Pulse: A Personal Journey in Cancer Research.* New York, NY: First Pulse Projects, 1998.

around it, while the outgoing current flows along the proteins of the cytoskeleton and crosses the cell membrane towards the extracellular matrix. Garnett theorized that an alternating current oscillating circuit exists within cells between the cell membrane and the DNA, which is activated during differentiation to initiate gene expression.

If this theory is correct, it means not only do cells use their electromagnetic properties to control gene expression, but also that an external field can influence gene expression. This topic will be extensively addressed in the chapter on research performed by NASA.

Moreover, Garnett hypothesized that the part of the DNA wrapped around protein structures, such as nucleosomes[4], can present electronic inductance, just like an electric coil. The current flowing through the DNA helix can manifest its own energy field thus creating an impulse that from the DNA interacts with other biomolecules like those that make up the membrane.

These complex bio-electronic circuits that are formed, could be used by cells, as antennas able to receive and transmit signals or information, both inside an organism and from outside. This last hypothesis explains how external electromagnetic fields, even weak ones, can influence the behavior of biological tissues.

Of course, this is not the only explanation of how cells and tissues can interpose with electrical and electromagnetic signals of an endogenous or exogenous nature.

- According to Smith and Best[5], since cell membranes are composed of dielectric materials, a cell behaves like a dielectric resonator that produces an electromagnetic field in the space around it. This field does not radiate energy, but allows the cell to *oscillate in resonance* and interact with other cells. This means that applications of certain frequencies with suitable generators can improve or interfere with cellular resonance and metabolic and electrical functions.

---

[4] *The nucleosome consists of a protein center made up of eight proteins, around which DNA is enveloped.*

[5] *Smith C, Best S. Electromagnetic Man. New York: St. Martin's Press, 1989*

- Prof. H. Frohlich[6] predicted that the fundamental oscillation of the cell membrane is of the order of 100 GHz and that the biological tissues have the ability to create and use coherent oscillations to respond to external oscillations.
- According to Ross Adey[7], the glycoproteins present on the membrane (glycocalyx), which create the cell lining, act as both molecular chemical receptors and *electromagnetic or electric field antennas*. This last function would allow the cells to scan incoming frequencies and then fine tune their circuits to resonate at particular frequencies. Adey also documented that cells respond constructively to a wide range of frequencies including extremely low frequencies (ELF) in the 1-10 Hz range that includes that of Schumann resonance. Adey and other researchers have claimed that one of the effects of weak electromagnetic fields is the *release of calcium ions* into the cell.
- Most of the molecules in the body are electric dipoles; the electric fields, if of sufficient intensity, can induce the molecular dipoles to an orientation along the field lines. So when a biological tissue is exposed to an electric field of suitable frequency and amplitude, a preferential alignment of the dipoles is established. The cell membrane contains many dipole molecules; therefore, an electric field can trigger a mechanism that alters the permeability and membrane functions.

In conclusion, it can be said that cells and tissues:
- *Have an electromagnetic nature,*
- *Generate their own electromagnetic field, which allows them to control and guide metabolic reactions,*
- *Can communicate with each other by exchanging information with electrical and photonic signals,*
- *Can communicate with the outside world by providing useful information for a series of diagnoses,*
- *They can interact with external electromagnetic energies, which can be both curative and harmful.*

---

[6] *Frohlich H., ed. Biological Coherence and Response to External Stimuli. Heidelberg: Springer-Verlag, 1988.*

[7] *Adey WR. Physiological signaling across cell membranes and cooperative influences of extremely low frequency electromagnetic fields. In: Biological Coherence and Response to External Stimuli, H. Frohlich, ed., Heidelberg, Springer-Verlag, pgs 148-170, 1988.*

Measurements that can be performed on a human body

It is well known that the most intense spontaneous biomagnetic signals produced by a living being are those emitted by the heart, measurable through an electrocardiogram, those of the neuronal activity of the brain in the central nervous system, measurable through an electroencephalogram and those of muscular motor activity measurable through an electromyogram.

In addition to these "active" signals, it is also possible to perform various measurements of "passive" electrical parameters that can provide very important information to indicate the state of health of an organism.

The most important that are known are:
- The measure of resistance, which can be performed with Voll's Electroacupuncture;
- The measurement of impedance, through Bioimpedanceometry;
- Non-Linear Diagnostic Systems (NLS).

Having knowledge of these topics is essential to understand how the human body can be characterized by precise parameters of an electrical nature and consequently how it can react when it suffers damage or when it is exposed to electromagnetic fields and their description will be useful for understanding a series of concepts that will be subsequently addressed.

Electroacupuncture according to Voll (EAV)

Electroacupuncture according to Voll (EAV) is a technique that by exploiting the electrical parameters of the human organism (in this case, the resistance) is able to make very useful and accurate diagnoses. It is somewhat of a link between traditional Chinese acupuncture, Western clinical medicine, homotoxicology and homeopathy.

This method consists in verifying, using the tip of the electronic equipment, the bioelectric state of the acupuncture points and consequently giving clarifications and information on the nature of a disease.

Using this process, the following can be evaluated:
- Food intolerance
- Disturbances or poisoning from heavy metals or environmental pollutants, or from abuse of medicines
- Allergies
- Geopatie
- Disturbing fields such as scars, teeth, etc.
- Energy blocks
- Chronic inflammation of the liver, kidneys and pancreas
- Migraine and other forms of headache
- Dermatological diseases, such as atopic dermatitis, eczema, etc.
- Dental diseases, gums and intolerances towards dental materials
- Cardiovascular diseases
- Tendency to chronic recurrent infections
- Chronic fatigue
- Gastrointestinal diseases.

In Germany around the 1950s the German doctor Rheinold Voll, an expert in acupuncture, used a device which measurements were made of electrical resistance of the skin on classic acupuncture points or on special points called Leber. Based on the electrical resistance that the point presented in response to an electrical stimulation carried out on the point itself, it was possible to know whether a particular organ or apparatus, or a part of it, was in a healthy condition or not.

Acupuncture points have the characteristic of representing areas of the surface of our body with a reduced electrical resistance compared to the surrounding areas. Through these points, it is possible to send electrical stimuli (as input), and to receive output signals from the patient himself. The equipment is practically an ohmmeter, that is a meter of electric resistances and the signals sent and received are therefore microcurrents of variable intensity depending on the resistance that the current meets through the body.

A few years after the development of this device, Voll made a discovery that revolutionized the very use of this technology. He realized that the value of the resistance of the measured point could vary if the patient was put in contact with homeopathic substances.

During an examination performed with this equipment, it was possible to test many substances (more than 10,000), consisting of germs, bacteria, viruses, fungi, insecticides, drugs, general chemical agents and phytotherapics, all in homeopathic dilution, to highlight those that managed to normalize the identified altered values found in the first phase of the examination. The substances, thus identified would then constitute the therapy. After more than 60 years, this method is still used throughout the world and has greatly evolved since its introduction.

The in-depth study of this method has provided an anatomical meaning and precise localization of most of the points (receptors) placed on acupuncture meridians, handed down by the Chinese tradition, demonstrating that in the body flow, bioelectric currents are an expression of complex energy phenomena. The finding that the equilibrium of a point that shows unsuitable measures, can be rebalanced with a homeopathic substance, has confirmed that the two medicines (the homeopathic and acupuncture) are essentially **Informational Medicine**, able to affect the regulatory systems of the organism, on hormonal functions, on the release of neuro-humoral mediators, etc. Therefore, a state of good health is obtained when frequencies, bioelectric currents and electromagnetic fields of an endogenous nature are ordered, coherent and in harmony with each other.

Bioelectrical Impedance Analysis (BIA)

As in the previous discussion, bioelectrical impedance analysis (BIA) is a method of measurement of electrical parameters of the human body, even if in this case, there is an emission of electromagnetic waves in the human body. The BIA consists in measuring the resistance and reactance in the human body and the subsequent processing of the data, in order to provide qualitative data regarding body composition, hydration and nutritional status.

In particular, once the basic parameters are set for analysis (height, sex, weight, etc.) with this electronic equipment, it is possible to determine:
- Total body water (TBW)
- Extracellular water (ECW)
- Intracellular water (ICW)
- Body cell mass (BCM)
- Fat free mass (FFM)
- Fat mass (FM)
- Muscle mass (MM)
- Basal metabolism related to cell mass.

The tissues crossed by an electric current, can act as:
- Non-conductors, should not be crossed,
- Bad conductors, which are crossed through a little current,
- Good conductors, are allowed to cross,
- Dielectrics, which retain the charges.

The meaning of the electrical parameters in question is as follows:

Resistance (R): it is the capacity of the body, or part of it, to oppose the passage of electric current (effect due to the dissipation of energy). It is related entirely to bodily fluids. Less water is present in the tissue (e.g., bone, lipids), the higher the body's resistance. On the other hand, the higher the hydration, the lower the resistance. The extracellular matrix has a lower electrical resistance than the cell membrane, so the electric currents will preferably be conducted through this extracellular space.

Reactance (X): it can be inductive or capacitive; the latter is that characteristic of the human body and consists in the property of storing electrical charges (due to the conservation of energy). The capacitive Reactance is what is in a capacitor, that electronic component that is composed of two metal plates, which is separated by a thin layer of insulating material (dielectric).

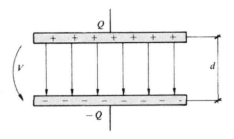

The cells contain different forms of biological condensers, which are made of an insulating material (the membrane) that are covered on both sides by fillers of dissolved minerals, which have the same properties as a conducting plate. The cell membrane and the membranes of organelles inside the cell, which are similar to the mitochondria, are biological condensers that have the ability to accumulate and store an electrical charge and therefore, the energy to be supplied when necessary (see Membrane Potential, cited above). Reactance of a body is directly proportional to the amount of active cell membranes, that is, to the body's cellular mass (cell density). The Reactance creates a phase difference between the current and the circuit voltage.

Impedance (Z): it is an overall measure of the body's ability to conduct the current. Mathematically, it is the vector sum of the Resistance **R** and of the Reactance **X** or the ratio between the induced voltage and the current injected in a conductive medium ($Z = \sqrt{R^2 + X^2} = V/I$).

Phase angle (α): it is the time delay between stimulation current and the alternating voltage applied in a conductive medium (in this case, the human body). The phase angle is expressed in degrees.

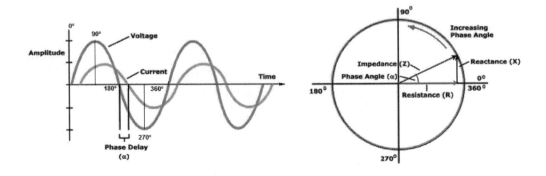

The temporal relation between voltage, current and phase is shown in the first figure above (on the left). The vector relationship between impedance, resistance, reactance and phase angle, is shown in the second figure above (on the right).

If we apply an alternating electric tension between two points of the human body, an electric current will circulate, which will depend on the impedance present between the two points. If this impedance were only resistive (i.e., Reactance = 0), the waves of tension and current would be perfectly in phase, that is the starting point and the trend, would be identical. If, on the other hand, the impedance were only reactive (Resistance = 0), the wave of the current would present a phase shift of 90°, which at the starting point would be at the highest point (crest) of the voltage wave.

The real situation is that the human body and the various organic tissues have both a resistive and a reactive component, hence impedance, which is a function of the electrical characteristics of the tissues and consequently creates a certain angle of displacement between Voltage and Current.
For example:
- The bone does not allow or almost, the crossing of the current (maximum resistance);
- Fat lipids are bad conductors for which they have a high resistance;
- Water is a good conductor of electric current (low resistance); lean tissue is rich in water;
- The plasma membranes (cellular) are dielectric, i.e., they are structures immersed in electrolytic solution that have the ability to temporarily store the charges. Therefore, they are the only body structures also equipped with a reactive (capacitive) as well as a resistance.

In conclusion, a bioimpedance analyzer, measuring resistance and reactance, is able to calculate the lean mass, the mass of the body cells, the total body water and the intracellular water. Studies of large populations have produced formulas from which the mass of body fat and body cell mass is obtained in kilograms and the quantities of water in liters for any combination of resistance and reactance measurements. These studies also established normal values based on age and gender and the relationship between these values and health.

The value of the <u>impedance decreases with the increase of the frequency</u> of the alternating current applied to the body. At the frequency of **1 Hz**, the current only passes through the extracellular fluids. At the frequency of **50 KHz** (the one commonly used for BIA analysis), the current passage is distributed equally between the intra and extracellular environment. To measure resistance and reactance, a bioimpedance analyzer applies a small electrical current (800 µA) to the body at a fixed[8] frequency of 50 kHz, using electrodes. Once the measurements have been performed, a microprocessor performs all the calculations related to the composition of the body in question.

It can be stated that:
- In the human body, low resistance is associated with large amounts of lean mass.
- High resistance is associated with small amounts of lean mass.
- Low reactance is associated with small amounts of cell mass. High reactance is associated with large amounts of cell mass (intracellular mass). Moreover, given that the reactance is of the capacitive type (capacitor from 500 to 1000 pF), a high reactance is an indicator of large quantities of intact cell membranes.
- Research on human beings has shown that the relationship between *phase angle and cellular health* is directly proportional, with an almost linear trend. A *low* phase angle is consistent with the inability of cells to store energy and is an indication of malfunctioning of the selective permeability of cell membranes. A *high* phase angle is an indication of large amounts of intact cell membranes and substantial cell mass. The phase angle reflects the relationship between the cell mass of the body and the lean mass.

The phase angles for adults can vary from 3 to 15 degrees, with normal values around 6 to 8 degrees. A low phase angle (low reactance) is therefore a sign of malfunctioning of the selective permeability of cell membranes and of low energy. A high phase angle (high reactance), is an indication of large quantities of intact cell membranes, cell mass and good energy.

Therefore the **phase angle** is a value of extreme importance and is proportional to the cellular health (regardless of the patient's weight); the results of this measure could be summarized as follows:

- A value in a range of **6 - 8 degrees** is an indication of normality, with intact cell membranes and good health conditions;

- A high value of phase angle (**values above 10°**), indicate large quantities of intact cell membranes, therefore high BCM (cellular mass) as in sports, or conditions of

---

[8] *There are also Multifrequency devices; the interpretation of the data obtained by means of a multifrequency bioimpedancemetry is complex because the total impedance and the cutaneous impedance vary, as well as the electrical properties of the tissues, with the frequency of the injected current.*

dehydration.

- A low phase angle value (**values below 5°**), indicate cellular decay or breakage of the cell membrane permeability, or an accumulation of extracellular fluids (water retention or edema) and may also occur under the following conditions:
- Oxidative damage of cells
- Sleep disorders
- Specific or non-specific inflammation
- Low nutritional intake or frequent use of processed food products
- Sleep disorders and sleep apnea
- Chronic infections
- Sedentary lifestyle
- Autoimmune diseases, chronic fatigue, fibromyalgia, arthritis, allergies and eczema
- Liver toxicity and/or stress
- Constipation, digestive problems and intoxication states
- Frequent meal jump
- Early aging

Non-linear Diagnostic Systems (NLS)

Non-Linear Diagnostic Systems are the most advanced and promising technologies in modern medicine; they include unique diagnostic tools based on spectral analysis of torsion magnetic fields in living organisms. It is the result of the research of a team of Russian scientists who in the 1980s invented a new and revolutionary system for the diagnosis of a large number of diseases and related therapies, called **Non Linear System**.

The operating principle of these machines is unfortunately not simple or easily understood since in this case we have to abandon classical physics and venture into the principles of quantum physics.

It is well known that quantum physics has revolutionized the concept of matter, which can be considered as composed of "mass, energy and information." It could also be defined as "structured, organized energy." The substance is in continuous transformation over time, with specific degrees of order and coherence as determined by "*information.*"

In this specific case, everything starts from the concept of trying to trace the state of health of a human organism based on changes in the torsion fields, a scientific concept that dates back to the early 1900s. The French physicist Eli Cartan in 1913 first proved that the flow of space and time possessed in it is also a rotation or spiral movement known as "torsion." This concept was then taken up and deepened by a group of great physicists in the Soviet Union of the 1980s, which began a series of research in the Center of Non-Traditional Technologies, sponsored by the state.

The torsion fields are generated by spin or a quantity, or quantum number, associated to the particles, which helps to define the quantum state. Depending on the orientation of the spin, both the left and right torsion fields can be generated.

In those years it was discovered that torsion fields have the characteristic of being influenced also by biological fields and so by the collaboration of physicists and geneticists, the applications of the torsion fields in medicine was born. Everyone has an extremely weak, low-frequency electromagnetic field, which in the event of a health problem may become distorted or incoherent. To implement an exchange of information between the machine and the human body according to the principles outlined above, it then became necessary to develop a *special trigger sensor*. The trigger sensor was developed using modern computer technologies and microcircuits, which was able to capture the weak fluctuations of the signals that evolved outside the statistical noise of the fields and converted into a digital sequence, processed with the help of a microprocessor and then transmitted to a computer via an interface cable. The human brain is capable of exerting an effect on this trigger sensor, but in order for this exchange of information to take place, it must receive a signal regarding the need to examine a given organ. The signal is sent to the brain via headphones, thanks to two coils contained within it, which emit waves at very low specific frequencies (below 10 Hz, close to the brain's Alpha or Theta rhythm.) Prompted by this request for information, the patient's brain sends a response that is thus captured by the *trigger sensor*.

The external electromagnetic fields then influence the magnetic moments of molecular currents, which lose their initial orientation; this causes a misalignment of the spin structures of the electrons located in the cortical neurons. It is natural that the most damaged tissues will have a more pronounced response, according to the logic theory of quantum entropy.

Some manufacturers of these devices use headphones that instead of using magnetic inductors use laser emitters to influence the patient's brain. The scan of all the organs that are examined, takes place in a few minutes. The device is always connected to a computer, which, in addition to displaying all the organs being scanned on the monitor, performs an analysis of the information received from the *trigger sensor* in real time. Once the scan is completed, the software performs a comparison of the data received with its own database, which contains reference parameters that take into account the main physical characteristics of the subject under examination (age, sex, etc.). In this way, it is possible to ascertain any dysfunctions or pathologies, the severity of the same and identifies possible remedies, both of an allopathic, homeopathic and phytotherapeutic type, etc. Furthermore, detecting the distorted frequencies may make it possible to send the correct frequencies to restore the electromagnetic field.

Since emotions also have their specific frequencies, it is possible to draw an emotional and psychological picture of the person, to investigate the unconscious traumas and to detect the state of psychological stress. A state of psychophysical wellbeing can be achieved by re-harmonizing the frequencies connected to the psychological state, releasing stress and tension and also acting on past traumas and on the conflicts that have given rise to the specific disease or problem.

It must however be taken into account that the analysis of the data highlighted by the scan, is not always easy to interpret, due to:
- Imbalances or old diseases,
- Diseases in the initial phase,
- Results that apparently do not have a logical link of communication.

Currently, there are several manufacturers of these devices that come from the original research group. Reviewing the most known and reliable devices, I find are only two that I would consider using [9]. Unfortunately, there are many clones available on the online stores, which might be confusing to someone looking to purchase one. The choice, even if it will probably disappoint someone, is not at all difficult. The original equipment is distinguished by the price (rather high, due to continuous research and evolution) and for the assistance that they are able to provide. All the others are almost always empty boxes, which use their database to show randomly generated data, therefore without any real analysis and reliability.

---

[9] *Among the best known companies that have continued to study and develop this technology are the producers of Diacom and Metatron. Naturally these names are swept up in every way by the producers of the fake clones.*

Effects of electro-magnetic fields

To understand how electromagnetic fields can interact with biological tissues it is important to know the main effects on cells and tissues. Electromagnetic fields must be considered not only on the basis of their intensity, but also as vectors or carriers of *information*, in fact the application of waves of even weak intensity *can be **high in biological information***.

The weak electromagnetic fields (electrical and photonic) can be bioenergetics, bioinformational, non-ionizing and non-thermal; they affect biological organisms, tissues and cells, which can be synchronized on specific frequencies. The answer is in function above all, of the right frequency before the amplitude and duration, producing great results when the synchronization is correct.

Effects of electromagnetic waves at low frequencies

At low frequencies, the electric field and the magnetic field must be considered separately; the effects of electromagnetic waves on an organism and in particular on a tissue are determined by many physical (frequency, waveform, polarization, modulation, exposure time) and biological (property of the affected area, dimensions, orientation with respect to the lines of force) variables and are modified according to the different characteristics of the organism, such as skin thickness, hair, hydration, age and sex.

At low frequencies (up to some hundreds of kHz), electric fields modify the charge distribution on the tissues and induce a flow of electric current while the magnetic fields, induce the circulation of magnetic currents creating a potential difference on the cell membranes.

Based on the studies and experimental data (obtained with in vitro tests or on animal, such as guinea pigs) currently available, the following effects emerge:
• Thermal,
• Alterations of the enzymatic activity,
• Modification of the calcium content in cells (transport of ions into and out of cells),
• Alterations of the cell membrane proteins and consequent modification of the ion exchange through the membrane itself,

• *Resonance* between the frequency of the electromagnetic field and some cellular processes, even at very low field strengths, it is the process considered to be more responsive to most of the frequencies used in Rifing. However, in this case the resonance is not to be understood as a destructive process, but as a means of amplification, which processes and restores the functionality of the cells in the re-balancing of tissues and organs.

Therefore, these effects are manifested above all as more or less explicit alterations of the cellular function, which will then result in results on the tissues and organs affected by the therapy.

In a recent study on the subject[10], while confirming that the exposure to low-frequency electromagnetic fields is a non-invasive approach for the treatment of various sensory and neurological disorders, it is admitted that there is still a limited understanding of the mechanisms underlying biological effects and potential targets at the cellular level. However, the results of the experiments demonstrated that electromagnetic stimulation has important effects on the responses of calcium ions on peripheral sensory neurons. Further studies, currently underway, will be necessary to further clarify whether and to what extent, electromagnetic fields can influence the different ion channels that contribute to the propagation of the action potential in sensory neurons. These ionic channels are expected to be inherently capable of specific conformational changes of the stimulus and their involvement will bring us closer to understanding how these processes could occur.

---

[10] *Acute exposure to high-induction electromagnetic field affects activity of model peripheral sensory neurons* - Published in: J Cell Mol Med 2018; 22 (2): 1355-1362

Effects of electromagnetic waves at high frequencies

When the frequencies are higher than about 10 MHz, the predominant effect is the thermal effect that is the heating of the tissues, which in any case will be proportional to the energy of the irradiating medium and to that absorbed by the irradiated tissues. Above 10 GHz, since the penetration depth of the electromagnetic waves in the tissues is inversely proportional to the frequency, the absorption will be exclusively dependent on the skin.

We will examine what happens to a biological medium when it is exposed to frequencies of the order of some GHz.

The principles of operation of a microwave oven can help us to understand the interaction of electromagnetic fields at high frequencies. The electric field essentially interacts with the polar water molecules, forcing them to follow its vibrations (about 1 billion per second = 1 GHz). These oscillations create a molecular friction that practically causes overheating of the food contained in the oven. With a biological tissue, things do not change. In the frequency range from 100 kHz to 10 GHz, the electromagnetic field gives energy to the tissues thanks to interaction mechanisms that cause the activation of vibrational states (the energy of the field is transformed into kinetic energy in the molecules); on the other hand, as already mentioned, as the frequency increases, the waves have more and more difficulty penetrating the vehicle. Furthermore, the transfer of energy also depends on how the electromagnetic wave is polarized and on whether it can *resonate* with a corpuscle invested (cells, bacteria, viruses, etc.). In fact, when the wavelength inside the fabric is equal to the dimensions of the corpuscle, resonance conditions can be created and in this case, the maximum values of the energy absorption[11] are obtained.

Another characteristic of high frequencies, is the ease with which the currents they generate can penetrate cell membranes which, being very thin (about 10 nanometers), behave like capacitors. In fact, a characteristic of the capacitors is that with increasing frequency, they tend to behave as a resistance of very low value, that is in practice as a conductor; the consequence is that the currents generated by the

---

[11] *"MECHANISMS OF INTERACTION OF ELECTROMAGNETIC FIELD WITH BIOLOGICAL TISSUE"* - www.progettomem.it

electric field pass through the membranes of cells and tissues more easily than the waves with lower frequencies and therefore can also influence the organelles contained in the cells.

These considerations remind us of the theories of Dr. Royal Rife. This eminent researcher, spent several years of his life identifying what he called "coordinative resonance" of different pathogens. In practice, Rife discovered that it was possible to devitalize microorganisms, if subjected to a precise frequency that could induce a phenomenon of mechanical resonance. Moreover, for what we are given to know, we cannot be sure that the frequencies identified and used by Royal Rife (in the order of hundreds of kHz up to some MHz), are actually the "fundamental" ones and not the subharmonic ones, but still of sufficient intensity for devitalization.

In light of the foregoing, it is now clear that to obtain appreciable results from a technology that uses these principles, it is essential not only to know the exact frequency of a pathogen (fungi, bacteria, viruses), but also to use the most suitable devices, so that these frequencies reach the microorganisms with sufficient power for this purpose. In conclusion, if frequencies become higher with greater difficulty an organic tissue, to obtain a *resonance* phenomenon it is absolutely necessary that the exposure times and the power at stake are adequate.

The harmful effects of electromagnetic waves

Nowadays, invaded by frequencies of Wi-Fi, cellular phones, radio links, power lines, etc., therefore from combined electric or magnetic fields or single ones, it is normal to ask oneself whether and how harmful the exposure to electromagnetic frequencies is.

The answer is unfortunately positive, but it is important to understand what the conditions that make these fields dangerous are and therefore the differences with the equipment for therapeutic uses. The conditions are quite common and can easily occur in everyday life, that is, *what can cause serious damage (such as cancer), is the combination of three fundamental factors:*

*A fixed **frequency** + a high emission **power** + very long exposure **duration***

These dangerous conditions can be found at any frequency, because it is not the frequency itself that is dangerous, but the fact that it is absolutely fixed, that is always the same, without any variation in time.

Few examples that can be commonly presented will make these concepts clear.

- Living near high voltage pylons means being subjected to *a very high number of hours* (think of the night hours) at a *fixed frequency* (in this case, 50 Hz), with *a very high electric field* determined by the high voltage of the power line and with an equally *high magnetic field* determined by the current flowing in the conductors, especially during the day when the maximum consumption is reached. Similar situations can occur, for example, in workplaces where there are powerful voltage transformers or large electric motors, but also in our homes when, with poorly installed electrical systems, the cables that supply a very high electrical load (e.g., a washing machine or an air conditioner) are installed in the bedroom, near our head.

- Spend many hours in a home or workplace, when a powerful antenna for cellular telephone or a radio repeater is installed on the front of the building (even in this case if the frequency is fixed and, even worse, it is very high). In this specific case, if it is pointed out that it is more dangerous to find oneself in the direction of emission of the antenna (for example in the opposite building), than under the pylon of the same (for example in an apartment under the antennas).

- Try spending many hours a day on the cell phone, without using a headset.

Think how many days, months and years you could pass under such conditions, perhaps without notice.

In particular, at high frequencies, the effects can be schematically divided into thermal effects, non-thermal effects, indirect effects and long-term effects.

Thermal effect: it is mainly caused by microwaves and, as widely documented by a large number of studies, is the consequence of the absorption of electromagnetic energy in the tissues, which is dissipated as heat. When prolonged exposure to these fields occurs, damage can occur especially in poorly vascularized tissues, such as the crystalline lens (cataract) and the testes (resulting in infertility and sterility). Damage of this kind can be subjected to power densities of at least 50/60 mW / cm2 with prolonged exposure times.

Non-thermal effects: they can also have long exposures at low intensity, i.e., below the threshold that can cause a thermal increase.
It has been observed that the interaction of high frequency electromagnetic fields with living matter can cause:

- A possible action of the electric field on the permeability of the cell membrane,
- Mutations in cells (both somatic and germinal),
- Consequences on the functions of the central nervous system,
- Loss of calcium ions in the nervous tissue and greater permeability of the blood-brain barrier,
- Effects on the cardiovascular system.

Indirect effects: when electromagnetic waves influence the correct functioning of electronic devices. The highest risks are with the pacemakers (problems of malfunction start to rise between 70 and 80 V/m, or 12-17 W/m^2), but also the electromedical equipment can be affected in their normal functioning (brain wave recorders, cardiac holters, hearing aids, monitors and meters of various kinds).

Long-term effects: although there is currently no solid scientific evidence or conclusive indications about the possible long-term effects of electromagnetic fields, it is known that the risks are mainly related to the onset of leukemia and cancer. Various studies and investigations have been carried out both on workers potentially exposed to radiofrequencies and microwaves (military personnel, employees of telecommunications industries, embassy personnel and workers involved in the microwave heat-sealing of plastic material), and on residents living in the proximity of telecommunications systems and in particular near radio and television repeaters.

The outcomes are not encouraging.

Hopefully, in the future, new epidemiological investigations and experimental research can be implemented so that it is possible to have more evaluations on the risks of short and long-term effects of exposure.

It is known that to counter these risks, there are several laws that are intended to protect the health of people and especially that of workers, but the precautions that each person can take, is the best means of prevention.

The combination of the three conditions described above, represents a situation absolutely never verifiable with Electrotherapy apparatus, Magnetotherapy, Rifing or any other device of emission of electromagnetic waves of the kind, above all because the frequencies used, never remain fixed for long periods of time. It is therefore deduced that these techniques are normally considered harmless; in any case, pacemaker wearers and pregnant women should be excluded from treatments of any kind.

With regard to Magnetotherapy and PEMF, the exclusion criteria must also include:
- Presence of benign or malignant proliferative diseases,
- Prostheses of material other than Titanium,
- Infectious joint diseases,
- Coronary insufficiency, hematological disorders and vascular problems,
- Organic functional alterations, psychopathologies and epilepsy,
- Some infectious diseases and mycosis,
- Thyroid hyper function and endocrine syndromes,
- Tuberculosis.

Application technologies for electromagnetic waves

The methods, with which the energies of an electric and magnetic nature have been and are still used, are innumerable. We will limit ourselves to analyzing the characteristics and the effects of the electromagnetic waves used by some of the most currently used technologies, in the range from 0 to the frequencies of light, therefore in the field of non-ionizing radiation.

The main methods of application and administration of these waves are listed below.

Therapies with light radiation

The light is the small part of the spectrum of the electromagnetic waves that we can perceive with the eyes. The nature of light is twofold: wave and particle, as wave is characterized by wavelength or frequency. The brain interprets the different wavelengths as colors ranging from red, with the longest wavelength (lower frequency) to violet of shorter wavelength (higher frequency).
The photons are the elementary particles of light.
Every day we can see how the frequencies of certain sounds or colors can influence our psyche (Limbic System), which in turn, through neuropeptides[12], can change in a positive or negative way our energy balance or our health and/or state of well-being.

The German biophysicist **Prof. Fritz Albert Popp** has succeeded in proving that the cells of any living being emit very weak light radiation called **biophotons**.

---

[12] *They are chemical messengers (neurotransmitters) of a protein nature that are freed in various areas of the brain or peripheral nerves and that modulate complex reactions related to behavior (mood, affectivity, sexual pleasure, aggression, instinct, pain, fear, etc.) and functions endocrine (sleep-wake rhythm, appetite, digestion, etc.) of our organism.*

The emission of electromagnetic energy propagates at the speed of light by means of DNA, which acts as a transceiver station, allowing constant electromagnetic communication, both inter-cellular and with the outside world (also long-distance).

Popp also discovered that healthy bodies emit very coherent bio-photon. While in poor health, bodies emit less coherent photons. The disease would be an interruption in the biophoton communication lines within the body due to parasites, viruses, fungi, pollutants etc. Furthermore, while investigating a particular light radiation with a wavelength equal to 380 nanometers, he discovered that it is associated with the repair of photo-phenomenon. If in fact a cell is damaged (and even almost totally destroyed) by the ultra violet light, it can repair itself alone in a matter of a day, if it is exposed to a radiation of the same frequency, but of much lower intensity.

In this category:

- **Heliotherapy:** it is a very ancient natural circulation, which is based on exposure to sunlight for the treatment of various kinds of disorders and diseases including: dermatologic, osteo-articular (activation of Vitamin D), respiratory, hematologic, circulatory system and mood disorders.

- **Light Therapy:** sunlight stimulates the serotonin and, especially in the Nordic countries where the insolation is very limited, this therapy is frequently used. In the field of chronobiology, it is best to administer light that mimics the conditions of the entire solar spectrum, through specific lamps, at a specific time, with a few sessions of ten minutes a day. The light which enters through the optic nerve, balances melatonin and serotonin and also regulates circadian rhythms, sleep-waking, improves mood, appetite and sleep quality. This therapy thus exploits the close connection between the retina and the suprachiasmatic nucleus (nucleus of the hypothalamus, which is where the biological clock of man is located) to reset the circadian rhythms that are out of phase in certain diseases, such as seasonal depression and the bipolar.

Therapeutic indications

This therapy has therefore been found useful for the treatment of depression, bulimia, sleep disorders and circadian rhythm, ADHD, dementia and altered sleep patterns, obsessive - compulsive disorder, headaches (not migraines) and cluster headaches, premenstrual syndrome, Chronic Fatigue syndrome, abnormal sleep patterns to work with night-day shifts and jet lag.

- **Photodynamic Therapy (PDT):** or Photochemotherapy, is an innovative technique successfully used especially in the treatment of cutaneous affections for the treatment of various pathological or aesthetic conditions, such as: acne removal, photodamage skin or injury due to skin aging, actinic or solar keratosis, pre-cancerous lesions and cancerous lesions (basal cell carcinoma, squamous cell carcinoma). The therapy is based on the irradiation of light at certain frequencies and the application of a photosensitizing substance in the form of cream or administered intravenously, which triggers an oxidative reaction, which causes only the pathological cells favoring the elimination and replacement with new cells.

- **Phototherapy:** is the use of light to cure a series of skin disorders (jaundice, psoriasis, etc.) and as a cosmetic treatment. The patient is exposed to specific light waves for a period of time.

- **Chromotherapy:** is an ancient therapeutic technique, that has natural origins, which studies the meaning of the colors and exploit its therapeutic properties to balance the chakras, relieve psychosomatic disorders and bring the body (mind and spirit) to a condition of well-being. Our body can absorb the colors in many ways (sun, lighting fixtures, clothes, food, etc.). The chromotherapy light irradiation is a very effective technique. The electromagnetic waves transmit energy capable of getting deep into cells, causing a series biological reactions, which will be described later.

- **Chromopuncture:** is the brilliant idea of German researcher **Peter Mandel** (early 1970s). It is a form of acupuncture that uses colored lights, instead of needles, which are directed on traditional acupuncture points to treat various diseases.

The therapy is also applied on some points located on the ear (chromopuncture headset) demonstrating that in some cases is more effective than the classical auricular puncture, given that the depth reached in the stimulation through the colors, is greater. These stimulations normally arouse a feeling of pain, although bearable, in the ear points that correspond to the energy area of the body affected by the disease.

- **LED and LASER Therapies**: the technology of laser light applied to the medical field saw its birth in the late 1970s. In the years following, this technique has evolved more and more. The use of this technology has expanded, including also LED light sources.

The main difference between the two light sources consists mainly in the fact that while the laser emits a *coherent light*, i.e., with all the rays in phase, the LED diodes do not have this characteristic. Both, however, emit monochromatic or single colored light, that is, at a precise wavelength, from infrared to ultraviolet (in the visible range, each frequency corresponds to a specific color and vice versa). In terms of frequencies, the visible spectrum varies between 400 and 1200 THz, which corresponds to a wavelength ranging from 800 to 400 nm (nanometers) or a comparable size to that of human cells.

In phototherapy and in many other therapeutic applications of monochromatic light, it appears that the differences between Laser and LED are not appreciable, since coherent light is converted into incoherent light when passed through the body. In practice, the therapeutic effect depends on the wavelength, the dose and the intensity, and therefore little or not at all on the coherence.

The absorption depends on the type of tissue that is irradiated and on the wavelength of the light. Light blue, green and yellow are almost completely absorbed by the skin surface. The red light is better transmitted than these are and the infrared is even better, at being able to achieve a penetration depth of up to 10 mm.

For therapeutic medical devices (mainly laser devices), the shades used are light blue, green, yellow, red and infrared, but especially the red/infrared light, between 900 and 630 nm, which are employed in most medical treatments. In this range of frequencies, the photons activate mainly the final vector of the mitochondrial respiratory chain (cytochrome-c-oxidase).

Mitochondria are organelles present in all animal cells whose main function is that of cell respiration and production of ATP, a coenzyme that can provide power to all cellular reactions and the processes of the body including, for example, the transmission of nerve impulses and muscle contraction. Mitochondria occupy about 10-15 percent of the volume of a living cell and they have their own DNA that comes entirely from the mother's oocyte.

Therefore, the red monochromatic light with a wavelength from 660 to 630 nm, acts by interfering with the mitochondrial respiratory chain of cells and more specifically on the enzymatic structures "cytochrome oxidase." This process results in an increased production of endogenous energy in the form of ATP (an increase of

150%) that the cell will use to improve its functions. From the therapeutic point of view, this will manifest itself as an improvement of the functional activity of that tissue "photo-stimulated" and then in a rapid restoration of its integrity. From this knowledge, derive many unexpected therapeutic applications.

The flow of light penetrating the tissues causes the biochemical reactions that induce several effects among which are:
- Vasodilation resulting in the increase in local heat, increase in cellular metabolic demands, neuro vegetative stimulation and modification of intra-capillary hydrostatic pressure (lowers blood pressure);
- Increased lymphatic drainage and activation of microcirculation;
- Anti-inflammatory, anti-edema and improvement of the nutritional state of tissues because of the increase in blood flow due to capillary and arteriolar vasodilation;
- Significant acceleration of regenerative processes, acceleration of the healing of wounds, increase in the potential of the nerve cells and a greater production of collagen and elastin;
- Increased production of endorphins and, consequently, treatment of acute and chronic pain;
- Care of trauma, injury to the ligaments, tendons, bones, nerves, skin, dental problems and infections (including herpes).

These applications are used in neurology, dentistry, dermatology (including cosmetic applications), physical therapy and rehabilitation (including the sports field). The light can be applied to any part of the body: blood vessels, skin, soft tissues, muscles, bones, brain and with LED devices and also to the eyes. The correct position of the laser probes or those realized with a matrix of laser diodes or LEDs, is important to avoid energy losses. Normally, the best position is perpendicular to the skin at the point of application and at a distance varying from 1-2 mm to a maximum of 1-5 cm. As already said, the light energy absorption primarily depends on the color of the light (or the wavelength of the beam) and on the constitution of the tissues that are invested by the radius (skin, blood, muscles, bones, etc.). The duration of the application depends on the energy (Joules / cm^2) radiated by the probe as a function of the depth of the tissue to be treated and the type of the beam emission (continuous, pulsating, modulated).

The light can be emitted continuously (e.g., to relieve pain), pulsating (e.g., to stimulate healing) or modulated frequency (e.g., for the application of Rife frequencies). Many authors consider the modulated laser light more effective in terms of therapeutic effects; some combine the continuous emission with frequency modulation by using the patient's reactions.

Finally, there is a wide range of studies (reflex therapy) that examines the effects of frequencies, with the stimulation of the points of acupuncture meridians, chakras, or trigger point (Dr. Nogier, Dr. Bahr, Dr. Reininger, etc.). The laser acupuncture combines the advantages of traditional Chinese acupuncture with modern laser technology. The correct frequency modulation of the laser beam on a point of acupuncture or meridians: stimulates the oscillation of the frequency of the meridian. This therapy is less invasive, less painful and safer than traditional acupuncture.

Electrostatic therapy

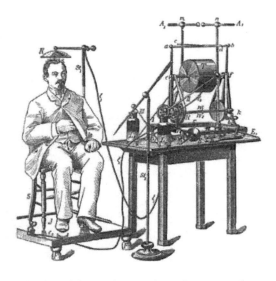

Among all the therapies that make use of electric fields, electrostatic is certainly the oldest used in clinical settings, given that the first clinical applications date back to the second half of the 1700s. The therapeutic principle on which all these machines are based is called Cellular Polarization.

It is the only case contemplated in this book, where the frequency is practically equal to 0. The therapy is performed by, applying a negative charge to the patient, which is electrically isolated from the earth and can reach up to 30,000V, by means of a copper handpiece connected to a generator of electrostatic currents (a little like the birds that are quietly perched on the wires of high voltage pylons, without risking any jolts).

The principle is based on the "dispersed capacity," that any element isolated from the ground, presents to the earth itself; in practice, the human body in direct current mode behaves like the armature of a capacitor, so that by applying a negative electric field to it, it is charged with electrons.

This therapy, through stimulation with negative electrical potential, solicits the minerals present, increasing the number of calcium and sodium ions. Serum potassium migrates to the inside of the cell, increasing its vitality, the movement of electrolytes normalizes and, tissue perfusion, improves. Another of the actions carried out by electrostatic therapy is represented by the maintenance of pH at basic (or alkaline) values, which is the optimal blood pH for cellular functions.

Although electrostatic therapy with constant electric field is the most widespread, there are also devices that generate pulsed fields.

Therapeutic indications

Considering the various stimulations that the Electrostatic therapy produces, different authors and producers recommend it as a means of great help for medical use, but also, it seems that good results are obtainable for type 2 diabetes, cell metabolism and stimulation of the microcirculation.

Electrotherapy or Electrostimulation

It is a technique known for at least 2500 years, when the Greek physicist Aetus, in about 500 BC used the biological electricity of a torpedo (70V), for the treatment of gout or electric shocks of an electric eel (Electrophorus electricus) for the treatment of headaches. The technique began to evolve in 1745, when the German physicist Aetus wrote the first book on electric therapies. The studies continued thanks to the French Jallabert and Marat who described the effects of electrostimulation on muscle contraction, to the Italian Galvani, to Faraday, to the French Ludec who designed an intermittent direct current stimulator. In the 1940s, the clinical application of electrostimulation became less popular due to the great progress achieved in pharmacotherapy, but was then re-evaluated in the following years thanks to its effective absence of side effects.

E-therapy consists in the application of alternating electric current, through electrodes placed in contact with the skin, to obtain effects of various kinds (electromagnetic, chemical and thermal), which are in turn responsible for therapeutic actions of the excitomotor type, vasomotor (vasodilatation), antalgic-sedative. It can be used to have a repolarizing effect on the cells (return to the resting phase), to obtain an increase in the arterial flow, increase the healing effect, the anti-edema effect (which reduces water retention), the anti-inflammatory one and acceleration of hematoma absorption.

Therapeutic indications
- In the medical field, for antalgic and anti-inflammatory therapy and for the

functional rehabilitation after the accident;
- In sports, for muscle strengthening and recovery;
- In the aesthetic field, for localized weight loss and lymphatic drainage.

In this category:

- (MET) Micro Current Electrical Stimulation or (MENS) Microcurrent Electrical Neuromuscular Stimulation: is a technique developed about 30 years ago.

The devices use a very low intensity current in the microampere range (10 to 1000 µA), with a long pulse width (0.5s). This slight current is below the threshold of man's pain and therefore is not perceived by the patient. In fact, the currents that the devices use are 1000 times less intense than those typical of TENS, even if with 2500 times longer pulse widths.

The administration of electric current in physiological intervals used by microcurrent devices, have different beneficial effects at the cellular level including: the increase of ATP of almost 500%, the improvement of the transport of amino acids through the membrane and the increase of cellular protein synthesis.

It is also likely that the transport of minerals through the cell membrane will improve, since microcurrent devices help to correct the electrical capacity (intended as a capacitor el.) of damaged cells. The damaged tissue begins to heal faster thanks to the increase of ATP or cellular energy and so the cells recover their functionality, while the tissues recover the normal conduction of electrical energy that allows the restoration of normal communication with the rest of the body through the connective tissue.

Several studies that were conducted with this technique had very interesting results. They were concerned with the intensity of the currents used: a stimulation of the MENS type at intensity of 500 µA in the epidermal tissue, which can increase up to 500% the level of the ATP (Adenosine triphosphate). Conversely, stimulation above 1,000 µA causes a decrease in ATP. The same phenomenon has been observed in the active transport of amino acids and proteins in synthesis.

One of the most accredited theories that explain the mechanisms of the action of microcurrents on damaged tissues is the following. As illustrated in the previous chapter, the resting membrane potential of a cell is

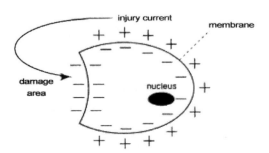

about -60 mV, with a positive charge on the external surface and a negative charge inside.

When cells or tissues are damaged (e.g., in case of wounds), the potential of the injured party from positive becomes negative and an electric current flows into the wounded area. This current is known as **"injury current."** The intensity of the injury current varies from 10 µA to 30 µA, so it is a microcurrent. The potential differences that are created and added, thanks to the contribution of all the damaged cells and the extracellular matrix, causes an effect similar to a battery that supplies electric current. The injury current triggers a biological repair and promotes the recovery of damaged cells and tissues in the living organism. Even more so, an artificially generated microcurrent can integrate and stimulate the natural functions of **"injury current,"** helping, thanks to the flow of ions that are created, to generate ATP, synthesize proteins and promote the reconstruction of damaged tissues; with these effects, the decrease of pain is only a natural consequence.

Therapeutic indications

One of the greatest advantages of MET therapy is the attenuation of acute and chronic pain and at the same time the reduction of inflammation, edema and swelling; it also increases freedom of movement, strength and muscle relaxation and accelerates wound healing.

It is exceptionally useful in:
- Soft tissue injuries, such as sprains;
- Decubitus sores, ulcers, wounds, post-surgical trauma and in the treatment of long-term residual pain due to post-surgical scars;
- For the treatment of headache, temporomandibular joint syndrome, neuropathies, arthritis and bursitis. Clinical experience indicates that this is an adjunctive therapy in earaches, sore throat, toothache, sinus congestion, viral or allergic conjunctivitis, post-herpetic neuralgia, post-CVA spasticity and compression neuropathy like the syndrome of the carpal tunnel;
- In preventing delayed muscle soreness after heavy exercise;
- To control hypertension, arthritis, Raynaud's syndrome, tinnitus[13] and post-anesthesia emesis;
- As a substitute for local anesthesia in dentistry and to control pain associated with

---

[13] Engleberg M, Bauer W. *Tanscutaneous electrical stimulation for tinnitus. Laryngoscope* 1985; 95:1167-73.

orthodontic treatment.

It has also been successfully treated with MET, the non-treatable pain in patients with carcinoma of the head and neck, even in some cases resistant to morphine. After only 10 minutes of MET therapy, the pain relief lasted from 8 hours to more than 3 weeks. The technique has been used successfully at the University of Texas MD Anderson Center [14].

Electrostimulation with microcurrents is also effective:
- In the regeneration of damaged tissues, ligaments and bone fractures (the analogies and electro-biological correlation of this technique with PEMF will be examined later);
- In promoting tissue regeneration and the production of new collagen and elastin (lifting effect - aesthetic use).

- (NMES) Neuromuscular Electrical Stimulation Devices:

the main purpose of this application is to create an excitomotive action on the muscle fibers in order to have a high stimulating capacity on the neuromuscular complex. This physiological approach to neuromuscular stimulation requires pulses of a shape similar to that of naturally occurring nerve signals, which have very short pulse widths.

In most cases the frequencies used ranged from 10 Hz to 120 Hz and pulse width from 70 - 250 µs, with the rest cycle as long as the work-cycle, to allow the dispersion of reactive hyperemia[15].

The current used can be of the Faradic, Rectangular, Triangular, Exponential and Kotz type. This last muscle stimulation consists in the application of sinusoidal current with a frequency of 2500 Hz modulated to "packages" of 10 ms (i.e., 10 ms of activity and 10 ms of pause), while the delivery occurs with stimulation period of 10 sec. and pause period of 50 sec. The use of this particular waveform guarantees a <u>moderate increase in muscle mass</u>, with an increase in strength developed by the muscle and a good tolerability.

The application of NMES, in addition to being the best known in the sports field, includes applications in the case of clinical problems of neurological, urological, orthopedic, rehabilitation, etc.

---

[14] *The Basis for Micro Current Electrical Therapy in Conventional Medical Practice - Journal of Advancement in Medicine Volume 8, Number 2, Summer 1995 - Joseph M. Mercola, DO and Daniel L Kirsch, Ph.D., DAAPM*

[15] *Reactive hyperemia is the increase of blood in a region following the restoration of blood flow after a period of temporary arrest.*

Therapeutic indications
- Increase in muscle strength and range of movement;
- Correction of spasticity contractures;
- Increase in sensory awareness and volitional muscle control;
- Decreased spasticity of the antagonist muscles;
- Re-education of muscle times with a series of muscle contractions coordinates;
- Substitution from the inhibitory effects of the nearby painful or inflamed area and from the painful joints on muscle contraction;
- Treatment for pharyngeal insufficiency to swallow (dysphagia);
- Neuromuscular stimulation in children with cerebral palsy.

- **(FES) Functional Electrical Stimulation**: is a technique used to produce contractions in paralyzed muscles, with the application of small impulses of electrical stimulation to the nerves that feed the paralyzed muscle. The stimulation is controlled in such a way as to generate functional movement. The operating principle is based on the use of electric stimulators of different types that cause the selective contraction of different muscle groups, in order to electrically stimulate the relative motor neuron.

Depending on the type of stimulator (internal, percutaneous, implanted), its positioning on the body of the subject and the intensity of the electric current it is possible to modulate, to a certain extent, the activation of the desired muscles.

Therapeutic indications
In order for the EDF to be effective, both the nerves and the muscles must be intact. In these situations the EDF can be used under conditions such as:
- Stroke
- Multiple sclerosis (MS)
- Spinal cord injury, T12 and higher (SCI)
- Parkinson's disease
- Cerebral palsy (CP)
- Head injury (HI)
- Familial or hereditary spastic paraparesis (FSP / HSP).

With these circumstances, the paralysis is due to a lesion of the superior motor neuron. The EDF can also be used in orthopedic conditions where muscle weakness is due to disuse or inhibition.

- (TENS) Transcutaneous Electrical Nerve Stimulation: the emission can be in continuous or packet mode (Burst) with a waveform that can be rectangular monophasic, biphasic, symmetrical, asymmetric or spike (very short pulse); the width (duration) of the pulse can vary from 30 to 400 microseconds, the frequency varies from 1 to 125 Hz and the current intensity from 0 to 80 mA. This technology is used almost exclusively to directly stimulate the nervous system by blocking the transmission of painful impulses and generating endorphins.

Patients are advised to set the current to the maximum comfortable tolerance, but the nervous system gradually adapts to this high level of current, causing a tolerance similar to that of chemical analgesics.

- (CES) Cranial Electrotherapy Stimulation: these treatments have been found to be effective for emotional or sleep disorders, but are now also considered an alternative treatment for pain. Two electrodes are placed on the ear lobes and a very weak electric current is circulated through the brain. The impulses stimulate the hypothalamus to produce more neuro-hormones (substantial increases in beta endorphins, adrenocorticotrophic hormone and serotonin).

From studies carried out by the US Air Force regarding acceleration of learning, it emerged that transcranial stimulation produces an increase in brain wave amplitude six times greater than when a subject is submitted to a placebo; the effect persists for a long time even after the end of stimulation. According to the researchers, stimulation would excite the cerebral cortex by increasing the response to sensory inputs and accelerating the processing of information in cortical circuits.

From magnetic resonance imaging, it emerged that the structural effects produced on the brain after stimulation persisted, even after five days. Specifically, the axons[16] are more robust and better organized after stimulation, even after days. According to the neurological studies carried out in the last decades, the formation of new connections between neurons and the strengthening of these connections would be the basis of the development of intelligence and memory. The effects produced by transcranial stimulation would confirm that structural changes would be produced by a series of alterations to brain tissue or to individual cells.

Therapeutic indications

Treatment of anxiety, depression and insomnia, acceleration of learning, brain injury, headaches, fibromyalgia, multiple sclerosis (experimental), smoking

---

[16] *The axons are large bundles of nerve fibers that connect the neurons together.*

cessation and opioid withdrawal.

- **H-waves**: are used to stimulate muscles and nerves, to promote circulation and alleviate pain and have been used to treat diabetic neuropathy, muscle sprains, temporomandibular joint dysfunctions, dystrophy sympathetic reflex and diabetic ulcers.

H-waves are classified as powerful muscle stimulators that produce rhythmic muscle contractions that increase local circulation and lymphatic drainage.

- **PENS Percutaneous Electrical Nerve Stimulation**: is the application of electric current through the insertion of a needle under the skin that is connected to the PENS device. The insertion of the needle is adjacent to a nerve. PENS is generally reserved for subjects who fail to obtain successes from the TENS units.

- **(PNT) Percutaneous Neuromodulation Therapy**: is a variant of PENS where up to ten fine-filament electrodes are placed temporarily in specific areas of the back, for chronic non-treatable pain relief or as auxiliary treatment in post-operative or post-traumatic pain management. In PNT, a doctor applies electrical stimulation through needles inserted from 2 cm to 4 cm away, in the tissues surrounding the vertebral column. It is thought that the electric currents applied through the needles stimulate the peripheral nerves. These nerves in turn can alter the activity of the spinal nerves that transmit the pain signal, resulting in pain reduction.

- **(HVGS) High Voltage Galvanic Stimulation**: it is characterized by an impulsive waveform (between 5 and 75 microseconds), voltage up to 500 V and frequencies in the order of 80-100 Hz for the treatment of acute pain and lower frequencies (8-20 Hz) for the treatment of chronic pain. The application of high voltage impulse stimulation is also used to reduce local edema. This treatment aims to reduce edema by shifting the charged proteins away from the edematous site.

- **(EAP) Electroacupuncture**: it is a method of stimulation of acupuncture points, through pulses of electric current at low voltage, through the use of needles normally used with this ancient medicine. Electroacupuncture was developed in China around 1934 and is still in use today, for example in chronic pain, spasms, difficult neuralgia or paralysis.

This therapy, a combination of electromagnetism with the theory of Traditional Chinese Medicine, can be practiced on all acupuncture points, including the auricular ones, those of the craniopuncture and the reflex zones.

All the equipment used in EAP are simple current pulse generators, which mainly use a particular asymmetric biphasic waveform (positive wave with a negative peak at a pulse width of 0.2 / 0.4 ms) and frequencies which can range from a minimum of 0.5 up to 5000 Hz. The effectiveness of this waveform has been clinically tested by a research group of the Shanghai Institute of Physiology.

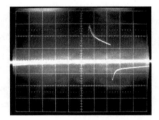 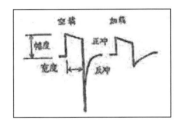

Each stimulator used in EAP has at least two outputs, and up to a maximum of six, each of which has intensity settings, as well as a frequency regulator and selectors for the choice of the waveform that is intended to be used for the duration of the treatment. Generally, in standard stimulators, the delivered current varies from 10 to 80 milliamps (mA), and the voltage can vary from 40 to 80 Volts, with the frequency from 1 to 100 Hz; the impulses can be continuous, alternated by pauses or wave trains.

There are many theories on the mechanism of action of electrical stimulation; one of the most accredited says that with this technique, the production of neurotransmitters, endorphins[17] in particular, is promoted, which are therefore responsible for the processes of analgesia, anesthesia, etc.

---

[17] *Endorphins, are opioid substances produced by the brain, classified as neurotransmitters, endowed with analgesic properties and are classified in: "Alpha, Beta, Gamma, Delta."*

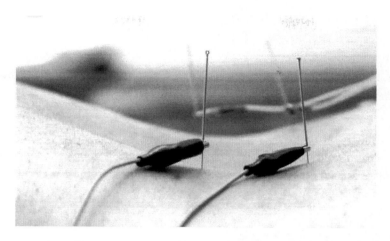

Some studies[18] compared the effects of administering frequencies from 2 to 100 Hz. With the low frequencies, an analgesic process is started mediated by the liberation of opioid substances (endorphins), while with the use of high frequencies the release of other neurotransmitters (serotonin[19]) is obtained.

In particular, with the low and medium frequencies, endorphins of the type meta-enkephalins, beta-endorphins and dynorphines are produced. As the frequency rises, (up to 100 Hz) it goes towards the production of serotonin. For example, a frequency of 2 Hz accelerates the release of enkephalin, β-endorphin and endomorphin in plasma, while that of 100 Hz selectively increases the release of dinorphine.

A combination of the two frequencies produces the simultaneous release of all four opioid peptides, causing an effect of maximum therapeutic benefit; this is the result of clinical trials in patients suffering from various types of chronic pain, including low back pain and diabetic neuropathic pain. It is therefore evident that an appropriate combination of frequencies can produce an optimal release of neuropeptides to have better therapeutic effects.

Some studies performed on humans have produced the following results.
- In a study on the effect of Electroacupuncture on low back pain, it has been noted that with this particular pain, low frequencies (2Hz) are more effective than medium-high frequencies (90Hz).
- In a study on analgesia for the surgical removal of the thyroid (electrically stimulated points 6PC and 4LI), the group that was given a 15 Hz electrostimulation

---

[18] *Information taken from: SCHOOL TAO BOLOGNA Acupuncture Course and Complementary Techniques "ELECTROSTIMULATION in ACUPUNCTURE"*

[19] *Serotonin has multiple effects such as: regulates the sleep / wake rhythm, the sense of satiety, body thermoregulation, platelet aggregation and stimulates the contraction of smooth muscles of vessels and bladder.*

obtained the most significant rate of analgesia, after 15 minutes.
- In 1953 in St. Petersburg, a group of researchers claimed that the ideal stimulus for the production of endorphins was 77 Hz.
- For nicotine addictions, a frequency of 10 Hertz was used, while for alcoholism or drug dependence it was reached up to frequencies of 100 Hz.

It has been established that analgesia can be achieved both by stimulating high intensity and low frequency, and by stimulating at low intensity and high frequency.

In the first case, analgesia takes some time to occur, but can last several hours after the stimulation stops.

In the second case, an almost immediate analgesia is obtained, but it is exhausted by the cessation of stimulation.

In general, the choice of frequencies can be made according to these principles:
- Use of low frequencies in the presence of situations characterized by energy deficit and for treating low areas of the body;
- Use of high frequencies in the presence of excess energy and for the treatment of high areas of the body.

Therapeutic indications

This technology is used to alleviate pain of any kind, but also includes all the possible applications of acupuncture, which strengthens and accelerates its effects.

- **Electrostimulation of acupuncture points:** is a fairly recent technique in which the electric current impulses are not applied through an electrical connection to acupuncture needles, but through an electrode with a spherical tip, directly on the acupuncture points. The devices are normally equipped with a handle, powered by batteries and almost always equipped with an acupoints detection function. The waveform used is almost always identical to that used in Electroacupuncture, or an asymmetric biphasic pulse with a width (or duration) of 260 µS. The current intensity can reach tens of milliamps, while the frequencies can be selected in a range from 1 to a few tens of Hz.

More sophisticated devices have frequencies suitable for the treatment of various health problems and electrode connection outputs, so that transcutaneous electrical stimulation (TENS) can also be performed.

Therapeutic indications

As in the previous case, the main use of this technology, is in the field of pain, but extends to the treatment of various other diseases. In most cases, these devices are accompanied by instruction booklets, indicating the acupuncture points to be stimulated, depending on the health problem to be treated.

Thermotherapy

It is a form of physical therapy that uses heat for therapeutic purposes. It is distinguished in exogenous thermotherapy, in which heat is transmitted from a medium outside the body (hot water packs, thermal baths, sand blasting, Bier ovens, etc.) and an endogenous thermotherapy, in which the heat is generated inside the body with the use of electromagnetic waves, which induces a temperature increase directly at the level of deep tissues (diathermy, radar therapy, etc.). In essence, endogenous thermotherapy creates fever, which is the body's natural mechanism for fighting diseases.

The heat is used:
- *In rheumatology and in pain therapy*, where the stimulus provoked comes into competition with the painful stimulus. The greater the heat exposure of damaged muscles, the less painful stimuli that come to the brain. In this way, it is possible to obtain great benefits with pain-relieving action (which is also obtained in tumor pain), anti-inflammatory action, against contractures, arthrosis pain, stiffness and muscle spasm.
- *In oncology*, where thanks to hyperthermia, energy is transferred to raise the temperature of the cancer cells in order to destroy or damage them. High temperatures can thus annihilate a malignant tumor without heating and damaging neighboring healthy tissues. Hyperthermia is indicated in all solid tumors. Furthermore, hyperthermia is used to increase the effectiveness of other oncological therapies such as radiotherapy and chemotherapy.
- *In the stimulation of the immune system*, due to the release of cytokines that stimulate the arrival of the leukocytes on the heated area, this contributes vigorously to the fight against the diseased cells.

Thermotherapy is therefore a valid method in the treatment of tumors and in the resolution of rheumatological diseases.

In this category:

- **Infrared rays**: they are electromagnetic radiations of a wavelength between 900 and 6300 nm, with frequencies at the limit of the visible band, below the red band. Infrared is produced by any hot body, with spontaneous emission. The infrared emission source is generally made up of carbon or tungsten filament lamps in inert gas, ceramic generators or coils, LEDs and Lasers. Their penetration power is limited (infrared rays A: max 5-10 mm, infrared rays B and C: max 0.5-1 mm).

Application procedure
Applications can be general or, more frequently, local. The lamp is placed about 20-60 cm from the area to be treated, with an intensity of about 0.25 W/cm^2; the exposure times increase progressively from 10 to 30 minutes maximum.

Among the biological effects produced, we observe:
- Thermal action, which indirectly gives rise to pulmonary hyperventilation, an increase in diuresis and a transient loss of weight due to the elimination of liquids;
- Local vasodilation with rapidly disappearing erythema and decreased blood pressure;
- muscle relaxation;
- Analgesic effect for reduction of conduction in sensory nerve endings;
- Increase in metabolism;
- Increased sweating, useful for the elimination of local toxins.

Therapeutic indications
Bedsores, Arthropathies, Muscular contractures and Skin trophic disorders.

With the advent of the latest technologies, Laser light is increasingly used to induce a local increase in temperature in the tissue, which can also be used for cancer therapy. The light energy is absorbed by the tissue and converted into heat. The light can be focused within thin optical fibers that can be inserted deep into the tumor mass or into natural cavities of the body, in a non-invasive way. Lasers are used both for hyperthermia and for thermotherapy. In this last case, we speak of Laser interstitial thermotherapy. Currently this treatment is mainly used in tumoral diseases of the liver, lung, pancreas, kidney, prostate and benign thyroid nodules.

- **Radar or Microwave therapy:** these devices emit electromagnetic waves in the UHF band, at the frequency of 2450 MHz (2.45 GHz), whose wavelength is 12.24 cm. The power of the generators is between 100 W in continuous supply up to 1500 W in pulsed supply.

The microwaves generated by a *magnetron*[20] cause a thermal increase inside the tissues due to the Joule effect (the electromagnetic energy is transformed into heat by means of the dielectric loss mechanism). Microwaves are selectively absorbed by tissues with high water content (muscle and periarticular tissues).

Application procedure

The patient must be in a comfortable position and remain stationary during treatment because it is immersed in an electromagnetic field. The energy can be administered to the patient by pointing the dispenser towards the area to be treated, about 10 - 20 centimeters away. The average duration of the applications varies between 10 and 20 minutes, every day, for cycles of 15-20 sessions repeatable after an appropriate interval.

Among the biological effects produced, we observe:
- Heating up to a maximum depth of penetration of 3 cm and low heating of the grease (the sensation of heat is less intense than the marconitherapy, but more pleasant and tolerated);
- Vasodilation and decreased sensitivity to pain (hypoalgesia);
- Sweating and hypotension.

The therapeutic effects of radar therapy are expressed in muscle relaxation (decontracting action), in a reduction of pain and in a marked trophic effect.

Therapeutic indications
- Skin infections (abscesses, acne, pustules)
- Traumas (pains, hematomas and localized edema)
- Chronic arthrosis, arthropathy, arthritis, periarthritis, lumbosciatalgie and cervicobrachialgie
- Fibrosites, bursitis, tendinitis and Raynaud's disease.

---

[20] *Magnetron is a type of high-power thermionic valve designed for the production of non-coherent microwaves.*

- **Marconitherapy:** shortwave devices for this therapy, use the HF band with a frequency of 27.3 MHz (wavelength approximately 11 m). The power of the generators is between 400 W in continuous supply up to 1000 W in pulsed supply.

Application procedure
Energy can be administered to the patient in different ways:
- Inductive mode, by means of a single electrode made of a flat helix conductor, on the area to be treated or with a spiral wound conductor around the region to be treated;
- Capacitive mode, with a pair of normally opposed electrodes, which are positioned in various ways on the area to be treated, two or three centimeters from the skin.

The patient must be in a comfortable position, as he must remain immobile for the duration of the treatment. The average duration of the applications is about 15 to 20 minutes, every day for cycles of 10 to 15 sessions, repeatable with intervals of at least 10 days.

Among the biological effects produced, we observe:
- Acceleration of cell metabolism;
- Immediate vasodilatation (deeper than IR) that lasts for about thirty minutes after the end of the application, prevalent in superficial tissues;
- Muscle relaxation and pain relief.

Therapeutic indications:
Circulatory alterations, Inflammations, Infections (sinusitis, tonsillitis, prostatitis), Chronic arthrosis, Traumas (stiffness and hematomas in the post-acute phase), Carpal tunnel syndrome, Herpes Zoster and Bell paralysis.

- **Tecar-Therapy (Capacitive and Resistive Electrical Transfer)**: uses electromagnetic waves in the MF band, at frequencies from 400 to 600 kHz. The power of the generators is between 50 W up to 300 W depending on the chosen energy level (low, medium, high) and the effects that you want to achieve.

It is a system for the production of endogenous heat, which will bring the biological tissues to high temperatures (43.5° C), and will manage to control, in real time, the intensity and depth of the heat produced. This method is widely used in oncology as illustrated below and is used in the treatment of some pathologies of the musculoskeletal system.

Application procedure

Using the principle of operation of a capacitor, the energy can be administered to the patient in different ways:

- Capacitive mode: with a pair of insulated or shielded electrodes normally opposed, one fixed (return electrode) and the other (active) with which a circular massage is carried out on the area to be treated. The targets of this modality are subcutaneous soft tissues and muscles;

- Resistive mode: with two fixed, non-shielded metallic electrodes, in which the organic tissues present between the two electrodes (bones, tendons, ligaments), which act as dielectric. The targets of this mode are bone, periosteum, tendons, ligaments and aponeuroses[21].

The sessions last approximately 30 minutes and twice weekly applications are recommended.

Among the biological effects produced, we observe:
- Acceleration of cell metabolism;
- Vasodilatation caused by heat;
- Antalgic effect, as a consequence of the increase in the threshold of sensory nerve endings, together with an increase in the elimination of pain-producing substances (bradykinin and histamine);
- Antifibrositic effect and reduction of joint stiffness;
- Stimulation of the immune system;
- Deep hyperemia (increase in blood flow) and reabsorption of edema and effusions.

Therapeutic indications
- Sprains, stiffness and post-traumatic pain syndromes;
- Contractures and muscle injuries, muscular pains and fibromyalgia and ossifying myositis;
- Tendinitis, tendinosis and insertional tendinopathies;
- Carpal tunnel syndrome;
- Arthrosis, lumbosciatalgie, scapoloomeral and coxofemoral periarthritis;
- Bursitis and fascites;
- Diseases due to venous and lymphatic insufficiency.

---

[21] *The aponeurosis or aponeurosis is the thin fibrous band that covers and envelops the muscle and goes on in the tendon, to ensure the bone insertion itself.*

Hyperthermia in oncology

It is a non-invasive therapeutic method, which aims to destroy solid neoplasms with a rise in temperature up to 42-43° C, through the irradiation of high frequency and high power electromagnetic waves (up to 600 Watts), by applying electrodes placed externally to the patient body and parallel to each other (capacitive mode), for a maximum duration of 60 minutes.

Deep tumors require equipment for Deep Hyperthermia that ensures effective penetration into the human body and work with antennas at frequencies between 70 MHz and 144 MHz or with a capacitive system at a frequency of 13.56 MHz. The superficial tumors can instead be treated with microwave devices with frequencies between 434Mhz and 915Mhz (ICT - Computerized and Thermostated Hyperthermia).

At this temperature, the tumor cells, which have a reduced vascular system and an altered cell membrane, cannot dispose of the heat, thus tending to accumulate it. This accumulation of active heat of the intracellular enzymes called Caspase will break up the DNA, activating the programmed cell death process (apoptosis). Furthermore, electromagnetic waves cause a depolarization of the altered mitochondrial membranes of tumor cells (with a very low membrane potential). The short circuit that is created between the two mitochondrial membranes induces the release of AIF (factor initiating apoptosis) and pro-apoptotic factors in general. Once the AIF is released into the cytoplasm, apoptosis can proceed independently, given the presence of the energy needed for the process.

The heat produced, affects only the tumor cells, while it does not damage the healthy cells that have a higher membrane potential; moreover, the normal cells being well sprayed by the blood can easily eliminate the extra heat received. Therefore, hyperthermia kills cancer cells in completely different ways than with other anti-tumor therapies and therefore it acts where the other therapies are not effective. Hyperthermia, besides being used alone, can greatly increase the effectiveness of other oncological therapies, such as radiotherapy and chemotherapy, thus reducing the side effects. In fact, when receiving hyperthermia and radiotherapy at the same time, the tumor cells, which are normally able to partially repair the damage suffered by irradiation, are no longer able to recover the biological functions and go to death (apoptosis). Several clinical studies have also shown that *low-dose radiation combined with hyperthermia* can be effective against cancer, compared to high doses alone. Therefore, combining heat with radiation can therefore produce effective treatments, while reducing the side effects of high doses (such as hair loss, exhaustion and nausea), hence, improving the quality of life of patients.

Instead of just using chemotherapy, hyperthermia acts by promoting vasodilation and therefore a more rapid and widespread diffusion of drugs in the circulation. Some tumors are treated with the triple combination of hyperthermia, chemotherapy and radiotherapy. Today, with advanced equipment and new knowledge it is possible to apply this therapy without causing any serious side effects and with very little risk.

The following tumor forms may be treated with hyperthermia: most solid deep tumors, superficial solid tumors (skin cancers such as melanomas, epitheliomas, superficial bone tumors and soft tissue neoplasms such as sarcomas), hematological tumors (lymphomas, leukemia, myelomas) and cutaneous and bone metastases.

Among the advantages of this therapy, we can list:
- Do not undergo surgery;
- Rapidity of the therapies: about 45 to 60 minutes per session, performed in the clinic;
- Absence of pain and therefore conditions of relaxation, during therapies;
- Absence of toxicity, as no drugs or radiation are used;
- Minimal damage to the tissues surrounding the tumor;
- Absence of side effects when used in combination with radio and chemo therapy;
- Improvement of the quality of life and increase in the survival rate.

The science of hyperthermia is constantly evolving, to develop increasingly precise and selective treatments in order to destroy cancer cells without causing any damage to healthy ones.

Ultrasound therapy

It is a therapy that uses frequencies higher than those perceivable by the human ear, applicable through a transducer that generates mechanical vibrations. They penetrate and propagate easily in an organic system consisting mainly of water (like the human body), giving energy to the system they pass through. You can reach frequencies of some MHz, but the higher the frequency, the greater the attenuation (and the lower the penetration depth). Normally these waves reach a depth between 1.5 and 5 cm.

The type of effects they create:
- Mechanical: micromassage and microconstructions with cell deformation, which translates into an acceleration of metabolism and cell reproduction.
- Thermal: The endogenous heat produced by ultrasound, has effects on vasodilation, superficial and deep vascularization and on the physiology of the neuron, which results in an antalgic, spasmolytic effect (calms muscle contractions caused by spasms) with anti-inflammatory consequences.
- Chemical: changes the pH and permeability of cell membranes, facilitating the exchange and migration of liquids; in addition there is flocculation[22] of colloids, elimination of gas, destruction of bacteria.

Therapeutic indications
- Fibrolytic effect: ultrasound has a marked ability to dissolve thrombus;
- In orthopedics: tendon, muscular or osseous pathologies, for inflammation, haematomas or fractures;
- Pain reduction: in sciatica, neuritis, periarthritis, tendinitis, tendinosis, tenosynovitis, epicondylitis, sub-acromial shoulder conflict, etc.;
- Disintegration of calcifications (lithotripsy);
- Aesthetic applications.

---

[22] *Flocculation consists of a chemical-physical process of a colloidal system in which the solid phase tends to separate, forming suspended flakes.*

Extracorporeal Shockwave Therapy (ESWT)

Radial shockwaves are high acoustic energy waves (therefore of a mechanical nature) that are transmitted with a probe, through the skin and radially (spherically) diffused into the body.

They are a sequence of single pulses of acoustic energy that propagate at supersonic speed in a liquid medium (1500m / sec in water), characterized by a rapid rise time (<10 nanoseconds), a high pressure peak (100 MPa), and a short life cycle (10 microseconds).

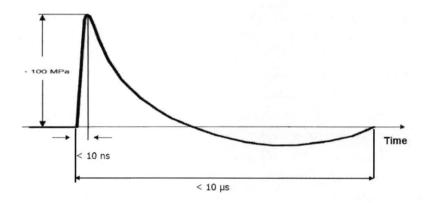

The technology comes from research in the military on damage to the internal organs of those who swam in waters where bombs of depth exploded. It was found that the shock waves produced damage that was concentrated in the interfaces with high acoustic impedances. Shockwaves were officially introduced into medicine in the 1980s for the treatment of kidney stones (lithotripsy - high-intensity waves); in the following years their field of use was extended to the orthopedic field, both for the care of soft tissues and bone tissues (medium intensity waves), and currently also for the treatment of erectile dysfunction. In the latter case, the shockwaves used were of low intensity; physical therapy was applied to the cavernous tissue, thus stimulating the circulation inside the penis and the gradual growth of new blood vessels, thus giving the patient a spontaneous erection that, unlike drugs, will last over time. The researchers believe that shock waves induce localized stress on the cell membrane that triggers a chain of events that result in the release of angiogenic factors (with an increase of nitric oxide, platelet growth factor and vascular endothelial growth factor). In addition, shock waves cause hyperpolarization of the cell membrane.

Application procedure

The technology used to generate the shockwave can be:
- Ballistic
- Electro-hydraulic
- Magnetostrictive
- Piezoelectric.

The applications are performed with the probe placed on the area to be treated, for 10 or more minutes. During the treatment, the acoustic impulses are created, at a variable frequency (about one pulse per second), while the power is dosed according to the therapy. In orthopedics, the therapy requires three to five sessions.

Among the biological effects produced, we observe:
- Angiogenesis (development of new blood vessels);
- Acceleration of cell metabolism;
- Regeneration and tissue repair;
- Multiplication and differentiation of stem cells.

Therapeutic indications
- Disaggregation of calcifications (lithotrissia) - kidney stones;
- Erectile dysfunction;
- Cellulitis and for body remodeling;
- Tendon and related diseases, even in the absence of calcifications;
- Pain, persistent edema and joint stiffness after surgery;
- Healing of chronic wounds, burns and diabetic ulcers.

Neuroacoustics

Breathing, heartbeats, brainwaves, vibrational frequencies of cells, molecules and atoms are all expressions of the rhythms on which organic life is based. If you hit a tuning fork, which produces waves at a fixed frequency by virtue of its physical characteristics and place it next to a second tuning fork, identical in shape and materials, this, within a short time, will resonate according to the oscillation frequency of the first. Similarly, also the human body and its organs, tissues and cells, can enter into resonance, or better, in bioresonance when they are invested by a well calibrated sound wave. This is why frequencies of artificial origin have a powerful influence on the organic ones: stimulating them, calming them, harmonizing them or on the contrary, creating discordances and disharmonies, as they always enter into resonance with the living biological systems.

Even with the biological systems, each of them, produces resonances with the other forms of life on the planet, creating various levels of harmony, but if we observe what has been studied in modern sciences concerning the interaction between psyche, body and artificial sources of sound frequency, is a very precise discipline that takes the name of Neuroacoustics and sometimes also called Music Therapy.

Neuroacoustics is a science that studies the action of sound on the brain and on the totality of the human organism, with the aim of producing a state of physical, mental and emotional well-being.

When we talk about Music Therapy the focus of our attention goes to the therapeutic effects that music or sound in general, can bring into our lives. On the other hand, when we investigate Neuroacoustics, the focus is on a set of experimental studies, which prove the relationship between receiving a set of frequencies in the headphones and the areas of the brain are activated as follows: how to reactivate the brain areas most vulnerable or inharmonious is the purpose of Neuroacoustics.

To do this, Neuroacoustics, uses balancing frequencies that tune the organs to their natural frequencies through a targeted stimulation of the auditory sensorial system; it is a process mediated by a large number of different techniques depending on the purpose, some of which are protected by copyright, as to exactly what happens in the record industry. The sounds at the various frequencies are mixed with the aim of solving various health problems, increasing the brain functions, getting rid of negative emotional states, create a deeper connection with our interiority and our spirituality, to reprogram the negative states that we assume daily and reconnect with the Self, the Universe and Nature.

The American scientist, **Thomas Budzinski** has invented many neuroacoustics programs, which validates his method to the world, the ability to treat, among other things, the syndrome of poor attention, alleviate alcohol dependence or eliminate epileptic attacks and schizophrenia.

American, physician and teacher of Psychoacoustics at the Institute of Human Sciences in Encinitas, California, **Jeffrey Thompson** is currently one of the leading experts in this field and is currently considered internationally as one of the leading experts in music therapy. He founded the Center for Neuroacoustic Research (CNR) in Carisbad, California, where the human body is studied in its psychophysical whole, following a neuroacoustic approach, i.e., the depth of the emotions, the areas of the brain and the parts of the body, which respond to the sound stimulation. Through his research he has developed a system of sound, which can be enjoyed with headphones, and which allow for individualized therapies that can work in harmony with special glasses, that are able to emit light pulses and are coordinated to the sound frequencies entering headphones.

His musical compositions are based on the profound influence that sounds has on the brain waves and are used by pranotherapists, psychologists, teachers and masseurs all over the world.

More recently, we got to know the brilliant work of the Russian-born researcher **Lenny Rossolovski**, who had the ability to recover, thanks to neuroacoustic therapy and developed an interest in this therapy that led him to the highest levels of this discipline.

The secret of the first neuroacoustic programs that were developed by Budzinski and Thompson, and later by other authors, was the use of the binaural technique, consisting in listening to two distinct, low intensity sounds on the two auricles. When a tone is heard with one ear and another slightly different tone is heard in the other ear, the brain reads a third tone pulsing at a phantom frequency which is the difference between the two starting tones. In other words, if a tone of 1000 Hz is submitted to the left ear and a tone of 1010 Hz is simultaneously submitted to the right ear, a third 10 Hz tone is processed and perceived by the brain producing an entrainment of 10 Hz. This technique, which can only work with stereo systems due to the impossibility of mono systems to produce two distinct sounds at the same time, has been surpassed and integrated by other newer and more performing techniques, which make the sound more complex in order to increase the effectiveness of modern neuroacoustics. Some examples are the triple sound modulation technique elaborated by Rossolovsky (Technique 3M), the mimetic background techniques that simulate the sounds of Nature or the spatial techniques suitable for reproduction on Dolby 5.1 systems.

This neuroacoustic programs are able to revitalize neuronal connections, to create new ones, to synchronize the hemispheres of the brain and to prolong life.

Therapeutic indications
- Removal of psycho-emotional blocks
- Increase in physical-postural balance
- Pain therapy, fibromyalgia
- Treatment of addictions
- Normalization of blood pressure
- Induction of a healthy and deep sleep
- Memory improvement
- Tejuvenation
- Energy balance of the chakras and rebalancing of the aura
- Synchronization of the cerebral hemispheres
- Entrainment of the mind on waves of type alpha, beta, gamma, theta, delta and epsilon.

Magnetotherapy

Magnetotherapy consists in the exposure to particular waves or pulses of magnetic or electromagnetic fields, which have therapeutic effects, induced by different modes of interaction between the magnetic field and ions, molecules, cells and organic tissues.

Magnetotherapy is a revolutionary and surprising therapeutic method born in the late 1960s by independent researchers, in the utter indifference of the scientific community, but with indisputable therapeutic results.

Currently there are thousands of scientific articles, also sophisticated magnetotherapy equipment used in major hospitals around the world, research and patents and also NASA (explained later), which attest to its effectiveness. Unfortunately, there is no standard of use and application, so every healthcare professional, doctor or hospital works according to their own personal criteria and experiences. Certainly, the thread that unites them all is the observation of the fact that many diseases or traumatic conditions, heal with a very high percentage of successes.

Classical magnetotherapy includes applications in which only a half wave, usually the positive one, of an electromagnetic wave is usually irradiated. The application devices are of electromagnetic type (coils, carpets, etc.) and they work by exploiting the magnetic field emitted by such devices with powers that can also be high (up to 3 Tesla) while the frequencies normally do not exceed a few hundred Hz.

The magnetic fields are able to induce, especially in the membrane and then in the cytoplasm, weak electric currents, of an intensity much lower than that involved in the natural stimulation of excitable tissues. The cells adapting themselves to the information transmitted by this electric signal artificially induced by the field, according to their functional characteristics, will have a series of different reactions depending on the type of signal and restoring conditions of energy imbalance. Furthermore, by acting on hemoglobin[23], it allows an increase of the concentration of oxygen locally. In fact, since the hemoglobin is ferromagnetic, it is attracted by the magnetic fields, applied in that determined anatomical zone, and then freeing the oxygen it carries, with all the benefits that follow.

---

[23] *Hemoglobin is an iron-containing protein found in red blood cells; equipped with respiratory function, able to combine reversibly with molecular oxygen, has the function of carrying oxygen throughout the body.*

Among the biological effects produced, we observe:
- Vasodilation;
- Oxygenation of tissues;
- Neoangiogenic effect: invigorates the walls of blood vessels;
- Analgesic effect.

In this category:

- rTMS (Repetitive Transcranial Magnetic Stimulation): it is a non-invasive brain stimulation method that uses a magnetic field pulse emitted by a TMS coil to excite the neurons in a desired position of the cortex. Frequencies in the 1-200 Hz range are almost always used. Single-pulse TMS has been distinguished from repetitive TMS (rTMS) because it is a modification of the first in which the magnetic field is repeated for a short time, allowing nerve stimulation during their refractory period. The multiple pulses that are transmitted in the rTMS are discharged through a coil using multiple stimulators; the devices are classified as fast rTMS if the stimulation is greater than or equal to 1 Hz and slow rTMS if the stimulation is less than 1 Hz.

The stimulation method works by the principle of induction: a condenser is discharged to allow a strong current to pass through a coil placed over the scalp. The coils used have a peak magnetic field intensity ranging from 1.5 T to 2 T on the coil surface.

Therapeutic indications
Used in the treatment of psychiatric and neurological disorders such as depression, hallucinations, Parkinson's disease, etc.

- High-frequency magnetotherapy: uses a carrier frequency (between 18 and around 900 MHz) to transmit wave trains at different frequencies. The intensity used by these devices is lower than the one used for the low frequency, but the results are the same if not, in some cases, better. It is particularly indicated for the treatment of diseases affecting the soft tissues. Even these types of applications have proven effective for pain therapy.
The high frequencies have proved to be very "flexible," at being able to cure many diseases, however, constant and prolonged exposure to the electromagnetic field is necessary.

- **Low-frequency magnetic therapy**:
These are apparatuses that almost always use a square wave where the Duty Cycle[24] is normally modified appropriately; the power can reach a few hundred Gauss, while the frequencies up to several hundred Hz.

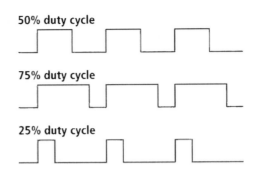

It is particularly indicated for the treatment of hard tissues and the delays of bone calcification (osteoporosis, fractures, post-operative recovery for prosthetic implants, etc.).

It is also indicated for pain therapy and in general to restore the correct functional balance of cells. It is therefore also effective in the treatment of soft tissues.

- **PEMF (Pulsed Electro-Magnetic Fields):** can be considered as a particular application of low frequency Magnetotherapy. These are devices that produce pulses of very short duration (from 100 μs to some milliseconds), often very high power (up to 3 Tesla) and normally very low frequencies (from 1 to some tens of Hz).

General Therapeutic indications

Some of the effects of high (HF) and low (BF) Magnetotherapy are:
- Antalgic effect (HF) (BF) and stimulation of endorphin production (HF)
- Neuroregulatory action on the hypothalamus, liver and spleen (HF)
- Regulation of intestinal motility (HF) (BF)
- Anti-aging action of tissues (HF) (BF)
- Improvement of skin metabolism (HF) (BF)
- Bacteriostatic activity (HF) (BF)

Also regarding the effects on bone tissue:
- Increased bone strength (BF)
- Improvement of osteogenesis (BF)
- Increase in mineralization (BF)

---

[24] *The Duty Cycle of a square wave is the ratio between the duration of the "high" signal and the total period of the signal; in practice it indicates the time in which the square wave has certain amplitude before returning to 0.*

- Increased production and deposition of collagen (HF) (BF)
- Increase in vascular spraying, etc. (HF) (BF)

Magnetotherapy is used for:
- Relieve muscular and rheumatic pain (HF)
- Accelerate the healing of wounds and sores (HF)
- Treat myalgias, arthritis, lumbago, sciatic, migraines, headaches and vertigo (HF)
- Accelerate calcification in bone fractures (BF)
- Treat varicose veins, phlebitis, vasculopathies, gingivitis, sinusitis, rhinitis, otitis, tendinitis and talalgia (HF) (BF)
- Cure all inflammatory states (HF) (BF): activates a vasodilatory process with the consequent arrival, in the inflamed area, of substances useful for healing
- Rejuvenate the skin by attenuating wrinkles (HF)
- Strengthen the body's immune system (HF)
- Dermatology: Acne, burns, phlebitis, varicose veins, skin diseases, healing of large wounds, fistulas and sores (BF)
- Infections: Tonsillitis, Otitis, Herpes Zoster, etc. (BF)
- Diseases of various kinds: Asthma, Asthenia, Cellulite, Hypotension and Rhinitis (BF).

Rifing

Rifing means the exposure to electromagnetic fields, characterized by precise frequencies and harmonics, by means of various transmission devices, are connected to a Rife Machine: i.e., to a frequency generator. It is a technology that takes its name from Dr. Royal Rife, who in the first decades of the 20th century, managed to identify the devitalization frequencies of some pathogens (of the order of some hundreds of kHz up to some MHz). Starting from this therapeutic approach, currently with Rifing we embrace a very wide frequency spectrum ranging from 0 to at least 40 MHz, with the possibility of covering most of the techniques described above, without limitations related to electrical parameters of any kind (waveform, amplitude, duration, etc.). In this way, a Rife Machine is able to perform treatments that cover all the applications useful for restoring health and psycho-physical well-being.

When used for treatment, a very common feature of these devices is to use (even in low frequencies), not a single frequency, but a group of frequencies that are applied in succession. This means that the advantages obtainable are almost always, far superior to other similar treatments, as better explained in the chapter dedicated to this technology.

In many cases the term Rifing, is replaced by other the names of other machine manufacturers, which are able to generate electromagnetic frequencies.

Therapeutic indications
- Any pathology caused by trauma or dysfunctions of biological systems or systems. The limits are established only by the knowledge of the exact frequencies for the treatment of the specific problem.
- Detoxification of heavy metals and various chemical substances.
- Devitalization of viruses, bacteria and fungi. Also, in this case the only limit is that linked to the identification and knowledge of the frequency of coordinating resonance of the pathogen to be hit.

Pulsed Electro-Magnetic Fields (PEMF)

What is surprising about this method of application of electromagnetic waves is the contrast between the publications of thousands of scientific articles from all over the world and finding that often, the official medical community virtually ignores its existence.

Pulsed Eletro-Magnetic Fields (PEMFs) are considered a subset of therapies with variable magnetic fields, which over time; as already mentioned, use apparatuses which, are capable of producing Pulsed Electromagnetic Waves and must be able to produce:

- Pulses of very short duration (around 100 µs),

- High rates of up and down variation, of the order of Tesla / sec, thus promoting impulses or gusts (intensity up to 3 Tesla),

-Frequencies up to a few hundred Hz.

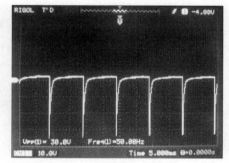

These are the main parameters that distinguish this PEMF therapy and differentiate it from the classic low-frequency Magnetotherapy. Unfortunately, however, in scientific articles, the authors tend to be inaccurate and classify as such, monophasic waveforms (positive half-wave only), biphasic waveforms (with both positive and negative impulses) and square waveforms with a very small Duty Cycle (with times of the order of a few milliseconds).

It therefore appears that in the scientific field, no clear distinction has ever been made. A strict classification should however consider PEMF as the only waveforms with the typical characteristics of the impulse and therefore having an extremely short duration and high intensity. Indeed, some studies have shown that short impulses enter the cells more easily, whereas longer impulses (typical of a square wave) are in some cases, less effective.

In practice, after examining all the main applications of electromagnetic waves, it is clear that each waveform (sinusoidal, square, impulsive, etc.) is able of producing different effects and results, even at the same frequency. This implies that the therapist must be very competent with all the techniques applicable with this therapy, in order to obtain the best results, in the shortest possible time.

The applications are carried out using coils of various shapes, depending on the application points and the power supplied. Each side of the coil is naturally characterized by two polarities: the north pole (magnetically, the negative pole "-") and the south pole side (+). For prolonged use, the (-) side may be the best to use since it is known to have a balancing effect, while the (+) side is known to have a stimulating effect. Many experts do not consider polarity with a pulsed magnetic field as important, since the aim is to create microcurrents in the tissues.

The pulsed magnetic field can interact with biological cells and tissues very broadly, succeeding in bringing beneficial effects to much pathology. In this way, it is possible to activate biophysical processes of surprising complexity and refined therapeutic efficacy, without damaging effects; in addition, pulsed magnetic fields are able to selectively activate biological processes necessary for the regeneration and repair of both functional and organic damage.

Effects on cells

In an organism, there are continuous displacements of electric charges, as there are different types of ions (H +, Na, K, Mg, etc.) that are in continuous movement between the cell membrane and the extracellular matrix. This movement of charges generates an electric field of very low intensity, to which a magnetic field of the same minimum energy is associated. Ion displacements are essential for the flow of information between the inside and outside of the cell, to activate cellular metabolism and for the balanced functioning of all tissues and organic systems.

As already mentioned, in a cell delimited by its own membrane, between its inside (cytosol) and the outside, there is a potential difference of about - 70/100 mV (membrane potential), which allows it to fulfill all its metabolic functions. A healthy cell manages to preserve the balance of the intracellular and extracellular concentration of the Na +, K +, Cl- ions, and is able to maintain constant the concentration of the fundamental nutrients (calcium and phosphate ion, glucose and protein anions).

When a lesion or disease manifests itself, depending on the severity, the cells begin to lose not only their functionality, but also their own energy. The concentration of oxygen in the tissues decreases, creating an insufficient production of available ATP, which causes a decrease in the sodium-potassium pump function. The result is that the voltage of the cell membrane can go down to -40 / -50 mV (which is already in the field of chronic pain and disease) in the tumor cells and the membrane potential drops to - 15 mV.

This premise will allow us to better understand the fundamental principles through which Pulsed Electromagnetic Fields act.

Magnetic waves are able to transport and therefore transfer electrical energy to tissues and cells; in particular, these overpeak stimuli increase the membrane potential, i.e., they initially lead the tension to high values and then re-stabilize on the starting ones. In biological tissues, even small but widespread alterations of permeability and membrane potential, can give rise to significant changes in cellular functions.

The final effect of pulsed waves is a gradual restoration of the membrane potential, which is carried out by activation of the ion pump Na-K; the powerful pulses of these very low frequency waves are therefore **able to bring the membrane potential back to the optimal values of -70/100 millivolt** *(resting potential).*

Of course, what happens in reality is a complex chain reaction, because in these processes, starting from the ions, there are chemical reactions on proteins, enzymes and other molecules, up to the involvement of the organelles contained in the cells, first among all, the mitochondria. It is therefore a question of bio-electrical and bio-chemical actions, closely related to each other. In this way, the impulse goes to act on the physiology of the cell, to rebalance it.

At this point, it is easier to understand how the characteristic shape of a pulse can be of considerable importance. We have previously stated that the generator must be able to produce an impulse (according to some authors, polarity does not matter) and not a classic square waveform. This electrical impulse must serve to create a temporary "upheaval" in ion exchange between the cell membrane and the extracellular matrix.

All this seems to bring us back, even by analogy, to heart impulses (the most complex part of the physiology of this organ). Only 1% of heart cells are specialized ones and are able to get excited. This excitement creates what is technically defined as a **depolarization**[25] of the cell, which creates an **action potential**[26] and therefore the birth of an electric current. Without going into rather difficult explanations, it is enough to know that all these processes of depolarization and repolarization occur naturally through a series of rapid ionic exchanges on cell walls.

We can conclude this topic concerning the membrane potential, with this reflection: the heart is the only organ that cannot get cancer. And, for a good reason, it is the most electrically charged organ in our body.

Therapeutic applications

The therapeutic action of the Pulsed Magnetic Fields, have a vastness of applications and effectiveness.
It is used successfully for:
- Localized inflammation
- Improve vasodilation, the development of new blood vessels (angiogenesis) and the oxygenation of blood
- Reduction of chronic pain
- Pain management and post-surgical edema
- Pain relief for arthritis and joint pain, fibromyalgia, back pain and ankylosing spondylitis
- Nerve pain problems
- Reducing the recovery time of sportsmen who have suffered traumas or injuries
- Delaying in the consolidation of fractures, stimulating bone regeneration, improving bone density, and in helping in the recovery of osteoporosis, arthritis and osteoarthritis
- The care of soft tissues such as muscles, ligaments and skin
- Patients with Parkinson's, Alzheimer's and Stroke
- Migraine, insomnia, stress, anxiety and phobias.

---

[25] *The depolarization of an excitable cell is the decrease of intracellular negativity, i.e., the decrease of an electrical potential of the cell membrane.*

[26] *In physiology, it is indicated as an action potential, the response to a short-lived event that reverses the electrical polarity of the cell membrane in the excitable cells.*

The studies and experiments[27] carried out so far have shown that PEMF with great intensity and pulse duration of about **100 μs**, have been effective for:
- Glaucoma
- Retinopathy
- Headaches - Horton cellular giganto temporal arteritis
- Tinnitus
- Mastoiditis (adjuvant in antibiotic therapy)
- Otitis (adjuvant in antibiotic therapy)
- Sinusitis, Laryngitis, Pharyngitis
- Dental abscesses - granulomas (inflammatory phase only)
- Osteoporosis of the jaw and paradontosis
- Herpes simplex of the lips
- Musculoskeletal disorders of the neck of inflammatory etiology
- Carotid stenosis
- Hyperthyroidism
- Flogosis of the joint capsule and tendons
- Epicondylitis
- Carpal tunnel
- Rhizarthrosis
- Herpetic and post-herpetic neuralgia
- Hiatal hernia (adjuvant)
- Gastralgia (alternative: high-frequency magnetotherapy in magnetic field)
- Hepatobiliary syndromes with obstructive etiology (alternative: high-frequency magn.)
- Fatty liver disease (alternative: high-frequency magnetotherapy)
- Tears of the intercostal muscles and / or rheumatic pains
- Herpetic and post-herpetic neuralgia
- Herniated disc and sciatica
- Coxarthrosis
- Gonarthrosis Venous disorders: Phlegmasia alba dolens (in particular thrombosis of the popliteal tract of the femoral vein)
- Phlebitis and thrombophlebitis
- Diabetic foot
- Achilles tendinitis

---

[27] *Marco Montanari : MAGNETOTERAPIA INNOVATIVA A BASSA FREQUENZA A SCARICA CAPACITIVA - published in 2017- http://www.fieldsforlife.org*

- Depressive syndromes
- Parkinson's and Parkinsonism

In the following paragraphs, some of these scientific studies will be analyzed in greater detail.

Pain

In damaged tissue, decreases occur in the amount of ATP, that in turn causes a decrease in oxygenation and cellular nourishment, which will hinder the functionality of the sodium pump, favoring the increase of tissue toxic substances. All of these metabolic changes are then perceived by the individual as pain.

Most of the therapeutic uses of magnetic field exposure include, among the effects, a reduction in pain. There are a number of scientific studies indicating that endogenous and exogenous opioid systems can be influenced by exposure to magnetic fields.

Some animal investigations revealed increases in pain after the exposure sessions. In contrast to these studies, further research has shown that exposure to magnetic fields has practically relieved pain. In particular, in a study[28] conducted on land snails, it can be deduced that the specific ability of PEMF to induce analgesia does not originate from a stress response of a non-specific magnetic field, but rather appears to be related to the *specific form of magnetic field pulse* (in fact in this study it is reported that two types of pulsed waveforms failed to induce analgesia).

Human research has revealed positive effects from exposure to magnetic fields. Surely, the effect is primarily due to a decrease in inflammation, edema and a muscle relaxant. Furthermore, the induced currents in the nerve fibers, act by blocking the passage of pain sensations, that can create endorphins and increase the activity of lactate-dehydrogenase in the exposed musculature (so, that conditions of degradation from lactic acid, will stimulates nerve receptors, which will then cause pain).

---

[28] W. Thomas, M. Kavaliers, F. S. Prato, and K. P. Ossenkopp, "Antinociceptive Effects of a Pulsed Magnetic Field in the Land Snail, Cepaea nemoralis," Neuroscience Letters, 222, 1997.

The regeneration of tissues

After years of studies and research on pulsed fields, today we can affirm that the phenomenon of tissue regeneration extends to all the tissues of the human and animal organism. Scientific publications concerning bone fractures and bone formation, cartilaginous tissues, nervous tissues, etc., grow exponentially and with the successes obtained, in addition to increasing the interest of biologists and clinicians, encourage researchers to endeavor new experiments and investigations.

In an autonomous way, the body uses its own bioelectrical characteristics to naturally produce electric currents that are involved in repair and regeneration. Several studies have shown that the endogenous electrical currents flowing in the body is not a secondary process, but in reality is a control system used by the body to regulate the healing of various organic tissues.

Musculoskeletal disorders

The use of PEMF stimulation in the clinical treatment of therapeutically complicated problems of the musculoskeletal system, unconsolidated bone fractures, failed joint fusions, congenital pseudarthrosis, cartilage tissue repair, arthritis, rheumatoid arthritis and fibromyalgia can achieve excellent results.

The overall success rate for these skeletal muscle problems probably exceeds 80%.
Hundreds of studies on the subject have explained, demonstrated and described as possible causes of success from PEMF stimulation:
- Increases in mineralization,
- Angiogenesis,
- Production of collagen and endochondral ossification,
- Membrane effects (such as changes in Ca's ion channel),
- Effects mediated by cytokines[29] (e.g., TGF-β, PGE2),
- Greater cellular energy through a mechanism where the repetition frequency of the pulses (normally from 2 to 15 Hz) leads to an enhanced production of ATP.

---

[29] *Cytokines are small proteins produced by various types of cells usually in response to a stimulus that can change the behavior of other cells by inducing new activities such as growth, differentiation and death.*

Bone healing

The first studies to stimulate bone healing with electromagnetic waves were obtained using electrode systems directly implanted at the site of the fracture (the MET technique was then used, described in the previous chapter). Subsequently, the use of time-varying or pulsed magnetic fields used, were applied with magnetic coils that encompass the limb.

The pulsed magnetic field, which induces a small electric field (of the order of several µV / cm) in the tissues, is responsible for the physiological and therapeutic effects. So it is the <u>electrical component</u> (induced), rather than the magnetic one that causes the main effects and reactions.

Currently, PEMFs are mostly used to heal bone fractures in non-union conditions (failed fusions), delayed union, osteotomy[30]. Several studies have shown that this technique can promote bone formation around dental implants and can initiate chondrocyte growth and differentiation, thus promoting the angiogenesis and endothelial release of FGF-2[31]. Furthermore, PEMFs improve the synthesis of proteins constituting the extracellular matrix such as aggrecan[32] and type II collagen. Therefore, the cellular mechanisms involved in these processes are different, including increases in growth factors.

If a bone is mechanically stressed, a potential difference is generated in it, which consequently causes the circulation of tiny electric currents (piezoelectric effect). This effect, together with a mechanical effort, was considered the mechanisms underlying the transduction of physical tensions (compression and tension) in an electrical signal that promote bone formation. It was thus theorized that the piezoelectric properties of bones and cartilages form the basis for their formation and maintenance. Therefore, the bones will have the correct endogenous production of electric currents to stimulate the primitive cells to differentiate into osteoblasts and chondroblasts. The electric currents created through the piezoelectricity are also necessary for the deposition of calcium crystals.

Once the electrical properties of the tissues are considered to be of proper importance, then therapeutic strategies that support the biophysical electricity of the body can be developed to enhance the healing of the diseased tissues.

---

[30] *Osteotomy is a surgical procedure during which a bone is cut to shorten it, lengthen it or modify its alignment.*

[31] *FGF2, also known as the growth factor of the base fibroblasts (bFGF) and FGF-6, is a growth factor and a signaling protein encoded by the FGF2 gene.*

[32] *Aggrecan, also known as CSPCP (Cartilage-Specific Proteoglycan Core Protein), is a macromolecule present in the extracellular matrix of cartilages.*

Currently the theory of piezoelectricity has been partially overcome and it is believed that the origin of the electromechanical transduction, is due also to electrokinetic effects (sliding potentials), however the facts do not change much in regards to the effects of these tissues when invested from electromagnetic fields. A magnetic field moves electrically charged particles, which create small currents induced in the highly conductive extracellular fluid of the tissue; the potentials that are created, can act as transduction signals that then promote bone formation (a similar mechanism of action also occurs at the level of cartilage, which stimulate the chondrocytes).

This explains the reasons why there are accelerated processes of bone healing. Moreover, according to some authors, the vitamins useful for perpetuating the process of normal cartilage and bone maintenance, i.e., vitamin D (in particular D3) and vitamin K, administered during the treatment of the affected area, will improve and accelerate the training of new bone tissue and differentiate the expression of bone from cartilage in the tissue in question.

In conclusion, although PEMFs contain both electric fields and magnetic fields, the bone remodeling processes seem to respond primarily to the *electrical field* component. The magnetic field contributes less benefit to the process. From this observation (confirmed by similar studies on MET Electrotherapy) it could be inferred that since the electric field produced is very small compared to the magnetic field that induces it, to achieve the desired effects in a short time, <u>it may be necessary to use quite high powers.</u>

Nervous tissues

Starting from the 1970s, after studies in the field of the locomotor apparatus, new research has shown that therapies with pulsed electromagnetic fields (PEMF) can be effective for the regeneration of nerves and myelin sheath. The implications on the recovery of spinal cord injuries are also staggering.

The most important growth factors that play a role in nerve regeneration are nerve growth factor (NGF), insulin-like growth factor (IGF) and fibroblast growth factors (FGF). Activation of the neural tissue by Pulsed Waves has also been noted for the improvement of cAMP[33] concentration, whose main function consists in the activation of an enzyme to regulate the trans-membrane calcium passage through the ion channels or by cascade, in bringing to the increase of the available glucose.

The experiments performed on animals, have given positive results on injuries of the median-ulnar nerve, sciatic nerve, peroneal nerve, peripheral nerve and of the myelin sheath.

The many successes obtained with nerve regeneration have indicated the possibility that the use of PEMF can be effective in the treatment of disorders of the central nervous system, such as multiple sclerosis (MS). MS is a neurodegenerative disease in which the myelin sheath surrounding the neurons is damaged and nerve conduction is slowed. In a dedicated study[34], patients found a significant improvement in the performance scale (bladder control, cognitive function, fatigue level, hand function, mobility, sensations, spasticity and vision).

Further evidence exists in the work of Sandyk[35]. This study describes the consistent improvement of a patient with degenerative progressive multiple sclerosis. The patient showed noticeable improvement when subjected to treatment with extracranial applications at a frequency of 2-7 Hz and a magnetic field intensity of 7.5 pico Tesla (thus a very low power). In this study, it is hypothesized that therapeutic effects imply the mediating of the pineal gland, which is known to act as a magnetosensor. This study demonstrates, for the first time, the <u>remarkable effectiveness of small intensity magnetic fields</u>, in the symptomatic treatment of MS and underlines the key role of the pineal gland in MS pathophysiology.

---

[33] *cAMP is a cell metabolite produced by the enzyme adenylate cyclase from ATP. It is an important "second messenger" involved in the mechanisms of signal transduction within living cells in response to various stimuli, such as those induced by glucagon hormones or adrenaline, which are unable to cross the cell membrane.*

[34] T. L. Richards, M. S. Lappin, J. Acosta-Urquidi, G. H. Kraft, A. C. Heide, F. W. Lawrie, T. E. Merrill, G. B. Melton, and C. A. Cunningham, "Double-blind Study of Pulsing Magnetic Field Effects on Multiple Sclerosis," The Journal of Alterna- tise and Complementary Medicine, **3**, 1, 1997.

[35] *Int J Neurosci. 1992 Oct; 66(3-4)." Successful treatment of multiple sclerosis with magnetic fields." Sandyk R*

In an article by the same author[36], "*Magnetic Fields in the Therapy of Parkinsonism*" the problem of Parkinsonism is also addressed.

Furthermore, in this case, an extracranial treatment with magnetic fields of the order of picoTesla was used and the conclusions are that in all the patients an improvement of the disability and cognitive deficits were observed.

Many disorders of the central nervous system, spinal cord and psychiatric nature (depression, mood disorders, etc.) have been successfully resolved, with a technique practically identical to PEMF, called Transcranial Magnetic Stimulation (TMS or rTMS).

Based on the consistent bibliography of research and scientific studies, it can therefore be concluded that all types of problems related to the back, scoliosis, low back pain, sciatic nerve pain, problems with the cervical spine, hernia or damage to the disc and any other area of the body, which requires the regeneration of nerve tissues, may be beneficial with these therapies.

---

[36] *Sandyk R (1992): Magnetic fields in the therapy of Parkinsonism.*

Conclusions on PEMF

Therapy with PEMF is a method that allows results, which are superior to any other type of therapy, provided that the following conditions are met: accurate diagnosis, selection of the diseases to be treated, use of suitable equipment and correct use of the same. When the waveform, frequency and amplitude fall under certain parameters and the duration and frequency of the application are adequate, research has shown that PEMFs are able to produce miraculous effects without side effects or risk of infection.

Considering the large number of pathologies successfully solved using this technique, it can be understood that PEMFs act at the cellular level to stimulate cell metabolism and restore the membrane potential without any harmful side effects.

PEMFs are a completely safe and natural form of treatment, proven in countless scientific studies with surprising results, which can bring benefits to everyone, even animals.

NASA's research on electromagnetic waves

In recent years, I have given several lectures and conferences on the therapeutic properties of electromagnetic waves. I have often said in my lectures: "*I did a lot of research on the web, just out of curiosity, to see if I found a single article, about how astronauts are treated on orbital stations for any health issues or diseases, since they stay there for many months. Well, I have never been able to find an answer. So I asked myself, how do astronauts treat themselves, if not with these methods?* "

At a conference that I organized, there was a retired doctor who had worked at NASA. At the end of my lecture, this doctor introduced himself and we started to talk a little on the subject. He confirmed that my statements and deductions were completely accurate and that NASA owns state-of-the-art technologically advanced and sophisticated electromagnetic equipment.

NASA has invested a lot of money into research on the therapeutic use of electromagnetic waves, including stem cell research. In a specific study, NASA first discovered that a specific electromagnetic magnetic field signal greatly increases stem cell growth, and later that same electromagnetic signal can increase the growth of more than 120 genes[37].

Thomas J. Goodwin, Ph.D., NASA researcher, in a scientific paper published in September 2003, "*Physiological and molecular genetic effects of time varying electromagnetic fields on human neuronal cells,*" reports the results of an experimental research, in which he studied the effect of electromagnetic fields on the stimulation of neural stem cells, responsible for the transmission of electrical signals throughout the body.

The aim of the study was to find out whether it was possible to stimulate neural tissue regrowth with electromagnetic fields and improve electrical conductivity between neuronal cells. The results obtained on a neural cell culture have shown that stimulation with an electromagnetic field has dramatically improved the re-growth from 250% to 400%.

---

[37] *Genes are portions of the genome located in precise positions within the DNA sequence and contain the information necessary to encode molecules that have a function.*

The study concludes with the statement that the bioelectrical and biochemical process of electrical stimulation of nervous tissues is now a proven and documented reality; this technique could be used for a number of purposes, including the development of tissue for transplantation, the repair of traumatized tissues and the treatment of some neurodegenerative diseases.

This system for the growth of mammalian cells within a culture medium, facilitated by a variable electromagnetic field in time, was patented on October 11, 2002 (United States Patent 6,485,963), with the title "Growth stimulation of biological cells and tissue by electromagnetic fields and uses thereof." In the "Summary of the Invention," it is interesting to read that to increase the growth of nerve cells and other tissues, a variable electromagnetic field was used with a square wave at a frequency of 10 Hz.

In the following years, other patents were filed concerning increasingly sophisticated methods and apparatuses, in which Thomas J. Goodwin is among the inventors.
The last patent is dated March 13, 2018 and specifically concerns an ionic magnetic resonance multiple chamber (AIMR) culture apparatus to enhance or control the growth of biological cells and tissues. The apparatus has various embodiments and may include an electromagnetic chamber for the culture system and a modulating device for producing ionic magnetic resonance frequencies, ranging from about 7.8 Hz to about 59.9 Hz. In one embodiment, the alternating ionic magnetic resonance frequencies produced, are about 10, 14, 15, 16 or 32 Hz and, optionally, resonances that oscillate between about 8 and 14 Hz, while the alternating ion magnetic resonance field can have a field strength of about 0.01 Gauss to about 10000 Gauss.
From the above description, we understand that it is an extremely complex and very promising machine. But what is clear, however, is that to obtain results of certain effectiveness, the electromagnetic fields used has a very complete series of variable electrical parameters that intersect and combine to obtain particular configurations, to be adapted and modified according to the culture.

If this technology is applied to *culture systems* for proliferation, growth, enrichment, conditioning, modification and / or aggregation of mammalian cells and tissues, how are the devices intended for direct *human applications* evolving?

Without doing too much research, one answer can easily be found in another recent NASA patent of February 20, 2018 (Pat. No. 9,896,681).

The invention provides methods that include the exposure of mammalian cells or tissues to one or more stimulation fields, variable over time with predetermined profiles, by modifying the amplitude, waveform, magnetic field, slew rate, drop time, frequency, wavelength and duty cycle. In particular, the cells or tissues of mammals taken into consideration are chondrocytes[38], osteoblasts[39], osteocytes[40], osteoclasts[41] and nucleus pulposus[42] associated tissue (it may also include cartilaginous tissue, bone tissue, connective tissue, spongy tissue, tendon and muscle) or any combination. <u>Gene regulation</u>[43] on these cells, tissues or bones can promote retention, repair and reduction of compromised cartilage, bones and associated tissues.

*Therefore, the use of an electromagnetic field can modify, enhance or control growth and specific **gene** expression of biological cells and tissues.*

This also means that even under normal conditions, cells use their electrical properties to control gene expression.

These statements are of enormous importance and thus give a completely <u>new and different explanation</u> from those examined so far. Without discarding all the interpretations concerning the effects on the cell membrane, ion exchanges, etc., reported in the previous paragraphs, it is finally clarified that surely *<u>the predominant effect of the Electromagnetic Waves is to stimulate the genes, i.e., the elementary units of **information** genetics that correspond to segments of DNA, capable of producing proteins.</u>*

The various documents that accompany this patent and the others mentioned above provide a detailed list of all the genes that are involved in different therapeutic or culture applications.

---

[38] *Cells suitable for the production of articular cartilage.*

[39] *Cells specialized in the production of bone.*

[40] *Mature bone cells; they represent the mature stage of osteoblasts.*

[41] *Large cells, equipped with many nuclei, mobile and specialized in the reabsorption of bone tissue.*

[42] *A gelatinous substance in the center of the spinal disc, which distributes the hydraulic pressure in all directions inside each disk under compressive loads.*

[43] *Gene regulation is the process that allows a cell to express a certain group of genes in one context and to silence others.*

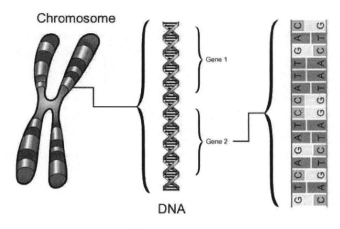

Genes

The apparatus for biomedical therapeutic applications, necessary to produce the stimulation fields, includes:
- A generator of signals or functions, able to supply to the target tissue, for a predetermined exposure time, an adequate magnetic field, characterized by a series of electrical parameters (frequency, wavelength, etc.);
- A means of transmitting the generated field, such as antennas or magnetic coils.

The system can take various configurations in which a <u>time-varying stimulation field</u> can be used in combination (or not), with a <u>pulsed stimulation field,</u> to perform various therapeutic applications. Each stimulation field is characterized by a "profile" that defines the various parameters; for example the Magnetic field can vary from 0.6 G to 200 Gauss, the frequency from about 9 Hz to 200 Hz, the rise time from about 0.125ms to 1ms, and the duty cycle from 65% to about 80%, with the square waveform.

Furthermore, the apparatus can operate for a predetermined exposure time from about 1 hour to about 1200 hours continuously or based on a time program. Deviations from the programs established for each type of application, can provoke different responses regarding mammalian cells, ion transport and therefore genetic and protein expression. For example, a stimulation field of a predetermined profile can be used to preferentially excite specific subcellular organelles within the cells in question.

In addition, the inventors have realized that the different stimulation fields can influence cells with regard to gene regulation, so as to produce a net **regenerative effect (anabolic)** or a net **repair effect (catabolic)** that can be used in combination with each other to design customized therapeutic applications.

In conclusion, by choosing the frequency, the appropriate waveform (e.g., a biphasic square wave or impulsive monophasic) and determined field strength, different results can be obtained; with these assumptions it is possible to carry out a series of studies or research, in order to obtain the best possible results in the **repair** or **regeneration** of an organic tissue.

Going into details, three examples shown in the patent documentation, clarify the above.

The waveforms used:

- The first, is basically a biphasic square wave, with a frequency of about 10 Hz, an 80% Duty Cycle and 10% Dwell;

- The second, is a single-phase impulsive wave, with a frequency of 15 Hz and a Duty Cycle of 30% (70% Dwell).

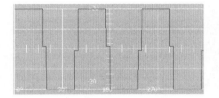
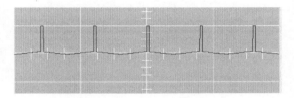

Square waveform   *Impulse waveform*

	Stimulation Field	**Waveform**	**B-Field Magnitude**	**Genes Regulated**	**Anabolic Effects**	**Catabolic Effects**
chondrocyte	First Stimulation Field	Square wave	0.059 G	2021	37	11
chondrocyte	Second Stimulation Field	Square wave	0.65 G	1097	**52**	3
chondrocyte	Third Stimulation Field	*Pulsed wave*	2.5 G	850	12	**15**
osteoblast	Fourth Stimulation Field	Square wave	0.65 G	2495	**87**	6
osteoblast	Fifth Stimulation Field	*Pulsed wave*	0.65 G	437	20	7

Summary table of the results produced by the experiments

1) In the first example, a sample of **chondrocyte** cells were used, exposed to a **first stimulation field**, characterized by a square wave and a magnetic field of 0.059 gauss. It was noted, that although the magnitude of the B field is rather low, the first stimulation field has involved the regulation of over 2000 genes. Furthermore, genes normally associated with a regenerative function (i.e., anabolic genes) are much more numerous than genes associated with a reparative function.

2) In the second experiment, two samples of chondrocyte cells were used, and exposed to:
   - A **second stimulation field**, characterized by a square wave and a magnetic field of 0.65 gauss;
   - A **third stimulation field**, characterized by an impulsive wave and a magnetic field of 2.5 gauss.

   It was noted, that despite the magnitude of field B is considerably higher, the number of regulated genes is much lower than in the first experiment (contrary to expectations). Moreover, with the second field genes normally associated with a regenerative function (i.e., the anabolic genes) are increased, while with the third stimulation field the genes associated with a reparative function are higher. Another aspect that surprised the researchers was the fact that the effects of the third field were very low compared to the others, even if a magnetic field of 2.5 gauss was applied.

3) In the third experiment, **osteoblast** cell samples were used, exposed to:
   - A **fourth stimulation field**, characterized by a square wave and a magnetic field of 0.65 gauss;
   - A **fifth stimulation field**, characterized by an impulsive wave and a magnetic field of 0.65 gauss.

   In this experiment, it was noted, that although the magnetic field is identical, the results associated with the fourth and fifth fields are considerably different. It is also surprising, as chondrocytes and osteoblasts, have had a different gene response even if exposed to the same stimulation field (the second and the fourth). This means that the same profile of the stimulation field applied to different tissues will lead to different results.

   Regarding the different genetic responses in chondrocytes with respect to osteoblasts, the inventors hypothesize that due to substantial differences in the total density of $CA2+$ and $K+$ ions in cartilage with respect to mineralized bone, the subcellular transcription signals are different when exposed to the same stimulation field.

With these results, which offer a new and precise explanation, with respect to all those read in scientific articles, it is finally explained <u>why each tissue presents a different reaction</u> when subjected to the same electromagnetic field.

We observed these phenomena several times, during the discussion on methods of application of electromagnetic waves (especially in Electrostimulation and Magnetotherapy), when, for example, it was found that with a specific application it is possible to simultaneously obtain:
- Angiogenesis (reaction on the tissues of blood vessels),
- Elimination of pain (reaction on nervous tissues),
- Restoration of the functionality of a tissue or an organ.

Another aspect of fundamental importance is the demonstration that different stimulation fields (variations in power and / or waveform) <u>can influence genes to achieve a regenerative (anabolic) or reparative (catabolic) effect</u>. The consequence is that with the right settings and sequences of magnetic fields, the effects can be combined to obtain the best solution based on the case to be treated.

Therefore, if we wanted to draw conclusions from this research, we could say that:

- *Each organic tissue, subjected to the <u>same electromagnetic stimulation field</u>, reacts with different methods, thanks to a different gene reaction;*

- *The <u>intensity of the electromagnetic field</u>, affects the gene response of the cells differently, depending on the invested tissue. It is important to note that the higher intensities do not necessarily bring better effectiveness or results;*

- *<u>Waveform, frequency</u> and other parameters of an electromagnetic wave, influence on the gene response of the cells differently, according to the invested tissue;*

- *Strong intensity pulsed fields can be more effective in gene stimulation, for **tissue repair**;*

- *Square-wave electromagnetic fields can be more effective in gene stimulation, for **tissue regeneration**.*

This research, makes us understand how only well organized and conducted studies, can lead to unexpected results and are absolutely unattainable with the classic methodologies that "traditional" medicine offers. The problem is that many researchers in the world, which study the effects of electromagnetic fields, unfortunately, do not have the resources of NASA, while for pharmaceutical companies, these researches are just a nuisance to hide or to discredit.

After the analysis of the latter patent, it can be stated that despite everything, the evolution of the equipment is directed towards increasingly sophisticated and at the same time flexible technologies, so that it is possible to program all the parameters that distinguish a variable Magnetic field in time.

NASA uses these technologies not only in space, but also to treat astronauts back on Earth. In fact, in a zero-gravity environment, astronauts lose muscle tone. Even their bone density is significantly reduced, so when they return to Earth, they are usually unable to walk on their own and must be helped by means of various kinds.

Furthermore, the healthy natural magnetic field of the Earth and its resonance frequencies do not extend into space. The consequence is that when the astronauts return, they usually suffer from fatigue, depression and many other symptoms. Therefore, applications of electromagnetic waves are effective for the solution of many different health problems.

Rifing

Rifing is a technology that takes its name from Dr. Royal Raymond Rife, a great scientist, researcher and inventor who, in the early decades of the last century, managed to discover an infallible method to devitalize pathogens (viruses, bacteria and fungi). Rife was one of the first in the world to use electromagnetic frequencies for therapeutic use and certainly the first to use this technology for the treatment of infectious diseases caused by pathogens. Today, Rife equipment cannot only apply the frequencies for disabling individual microorganisms (killing frequencies), but also an immense number of frequencies suitable for health restoration (healing), detoxification (detox), and the application of active ingredients.

The modern concept of Rifing is the use of any electromagnetic frequency able to provide a benefit in health and/or well-being. The frequencies available on the generators have a range from 0 to some tens of MHz, able to solve, almost always, a huge number of health problems (from mental problems to even rare or serious diseases). This technology is currently used by experimenters in most countries.

Very few countries allow formal use. However, Rifing offers the most extensive and complete application of electromagnetic waves for therapeutic purposes.

Dr. Royal Raymond Rife

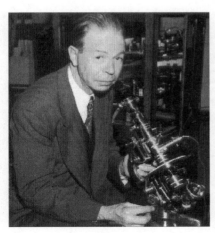

Royal Raymond Rife was born on May 16, 1888, in the state of Nebraska, by Royal Raymond Rife senior of Ohio and Ida May Cheney of Creston, Iowa.

From a young age, he devoted all his interests in the field of bacteriology. He worked hard in this field and photographed many species of microorganisms for the University of Heidelberg.

Thanks to the important contributions that Rife provided to the University, he was awarded an honorary doctorate in parasitology in 1914.

Since his studies on bacteria necessitated frequent use of microscopes, Dr. Rife developed a propensity for optics and began studies in this area. From 1915 to 1920, Rife worked in his private laboratory, identifying and classifying the microorganisms that cause many diseases. By the end of 1920, he had begun to work on cancer, but the limits of the microscopes available at this time hindered him in the discovery of the viral cause of disease. In fact, standard search microscopes built with optical lenses, like those manufactured today, could only enlarge a microorganism up to 2,500 times. Rife felt that with this limitation, he could never discover the true cause of many illnesses. In 1920-21 Rife built his first microscope; the famous "Universal Microscope," which was a thousand times more powerful than other traditional microscopes. His microscope used monochromatic light frequencies and quartz prisms instead of electron beams, which kill microbes. Rife was the first man to observe microorganisms without killing them.

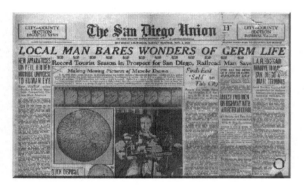

By 1938, Rife had built another four models of microscopes, each more precise and powerful than the one before, finally reaching up to 60,000 X magnifications. For the first time in history, photographs and film footage was taken of viruses and bacteria. (See the "The San Diego Union" news article).

It was in those years that Rife began to work using instruments capable of delivering electromagnetic frequencies. Rife wondered: "What would happen if I subjected these micro-organisms to different electrical frequencies?" With this revolutionary idea, he began to gather all the necessary tools such as standard research microscopes, electronic generators capable of producing the high frequencies with which he would work, bacteriological test tubes and instruments, guinea pig cages and other animals, machines for photographing species and additional equipment to build his own models.

Between 1921 and 1922, he built the first machine capable of delivering electromagnetic frequencies, the Rife Ray 1. Rife was assisted by Lee DeForest, the father of modern electronic tubes, which gave an important contribution to the first radio technology.

In 1933, he began working with Philip Hoyland, who lived in nearby Atladena, California. Hoyland helped Rife to build equipment, equipped with a ray tube that is a kind of plasma antenna consisting of a lamp filled with helium, powered by a very high voltage and driven by precise radiofrequencies.

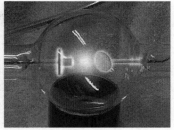

Both in the experiments performed in the laboratory and directly on the persons in care, Rife used this device to emit the frequencies capable of devitalizing the microbes by resonating them with electromagnetic waves.

Hoyland built most of the first machines, and in 1938 partnered with Royal Rife, to form Beam Rays Inc. This company produced the Rife Ray 5 or Beam Ray, until it became bankrupt a few years later after a series of vicissitudes and judicial problems.

Through arduous experimentation and looking through the microscopes of his invention while applying different frequencies, Dr. Rife discovered that it was possible in this way to devitalize these microorganisms. In fact, to determine which frequency would have killed a particular microorganism, it was absolutely essential to be able to observe them while they were alive, so that they could see the effect in real time.

His work was based on a basic principle called "coordinative resonance." To explain this principle, one could take as an example that of two tuning forks set to an absolute value: the moment one is stimulated, the other resounds. He thought, therefore, that with the stimulation of an electronic frequency able to pass through the tissues of the body, it was possible to devitalize a bacterium, <u>without damaging in any way the organs or the cells invested</u>, which instead have much higher resonance frequencies.

Rife described how he managed to find all the frequencies capable of killing the various microorganisms. As a crystal glass breaks if invested by its resonance frequency, in the same way the pathogens can be devitalized once their specific frequency has been identified.

So these electromagnetic waves, showed to possess the property of devitalizing or "killing" the microorganisms if invested by the exact resonance frequency (different for each organism). To discover the exact frequency of a pathogen, Rife with infinite patience observed the reactions under the microscope, varying from time to time the frequency of his equipment, until he found the desired effects.

Rife called the precise frequency able to kill a microorganism, **MOR** (Mortal Oscillatory Rate).

In 1922, Rife began to study a way to identify and destroy the viruses that caused cancer. His research on cancer took him ten years later, in 1932, to isolate the responsible pathogen that he called simply the BX virus.

In opposition to established medical theories, Rife in 1953 affirmed, that: "*This BX virus can easily turn into different forms during its life cycle according to the environment in which it grew up.*" Thus, its characteristic is pleomorphism (passage to different forms), causing different diseases depending on the stage of its development in the organism.

Another notable discovery was the PH-factor (acid-basic equilibrium). Rife declared that with a neutral PH, he could not produce any culture. On the contrary, with a basic or acid PH, it was able to produce a culture of microorganisms. Therefore, on the basis of this information, Dr. Rife came to the conclusion that as long as the human body is able to maintain the PH of the different organic systems in the right and natural equilibrium, it becomes impossible for a disease to develop.

After conducting thousands of experiments on infected cultures and animals, Rife was joined by some of the most prestigious doctors in the country, who financed him and used his equipment on men, with positive results.

In 1931 two people provided the maximum professional support to Dr. Rife: Dr. Arthur I. Kendall, director of medical research at the Northwestern University Medical School of Illinois and Dr. Milbank Johnson, member of the board of directors at Pasadena Hospital in California, very influential in Los Angeles medical circles.

Dr. Kendall had invented a protein culture medium, which he called "K-Medium," which allowed a bacterium to remain isolated and to continue reproducing. This became a very important support for Rife's experiments. Rife, Kendall and other scientists demonstrated that it was possible to grow bacteria artificially.

The technical discovery that leads to cancer treatment was published in the journal Science in 1931.

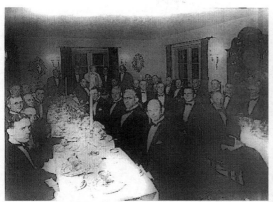After the successes obtained by Rife and Kendall, Dr. Milbank Johnson on November 20, 1931 organized a dinner in his Pasadena estate in honor of the two men, so that the discoveries could be announced and discussed. Forty-four of the most prominent doctors, pathologists and bacteriologists in Los Angeles took part in this historic event advertised as *"the end of all diseases."* Among those present were Dr. Alvin G. Ford, who 20 years later claimed to know little about Rife and his findings and Dr. George Dock who worked at the University of California Special Research Committee of the South, first supervisor of clinical work, later among opponents of Rife.

In 1934, Dr. Johnson began the first successful trials at the Jolla Clinic in California, on a series of patients with cancer and tuberculosis. In this hospital the first clinical cancer work was started, established under a special committee of the Medical Research of the University of Southern California, under the supervision of Johnson himself. The trial involved 16 terminal cancer patients. After 3 months, 14 of these desperate cases were declared as clinically healed by the staff of five doctors (Dr. Alvin G. Ford was the pathologist of the group), after another 130 days, following a change introduced in the treatment, even the last two patients healed. The treatments consisted in the application of electromagnetic waves for duration of 180 seconds, using a Rife Ray 3 set on the deadly frequency for cancer "BX," at intervals of 3 days. It was found that this time spent between two treatments, led to better results than the cases treated daily. In this way, the lymphatic system was given the opportunity to absorb and eliminate the toxic residues produced by dead microbes. The application of electromagnetic waves did not cause the body temperature to rise, nor were special diets given during the entire clinical treatment.

The results of this study showed that the cancer was caused by microorganisms and that such pathogens could be painlessly destroyed and finally that this disease could be cured.

In the years following the clinical success of 1934, the technology and curative treatment of cancer patients with Rife Ray, were discussed in medical conferences and data released in a medical journal.

In 1935, Dr. Johnson continued trials with a new machine installed at the Santa Fe Hospital in Los Angeles. In 1936, Johnson realized that Rife needed a new workshop to continue his work and, thanks to the help of some friends, he found the funds for the construction of a new and comfortable structure. In October-November of the same year, Dr. Johnson began using a Ray Machine in the Pasadena Home for the Aged clinic, reporting that he achieved excellent results.

Unfortunately, Dr. Johnson, a sufferer of heart, died in October 1944, while he was preparing a press release on the successes obtained with these machines.

In an article dated May 6, 1938 in the Evening Tribune, Rife, through a reporter, reported that he had experienced electrical stimulation on various microorganisms and that he had noticed the individual differences in the chemical constituents of the diseased organisms and had observed the specifications of the electrical characteristics and the polarities in the organisms.

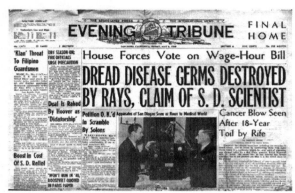

In 1939, his device was declared illegal and most of the 44 doctors who had acclaimed him eight years earlier, denied ever having met him. Some incidents such as the destruction of his laboratory, the killing of some people close to him and the destruction of all the documentation in their possession convinced Rife to put an end to his research.

Rife with his machines, successfully treated hundreds of patients who were diagnosed with incurable cancer and he received 14 awards and an honorary doctorate from the University of Heidelberg. All this occurred without the use of poisonous medicines, invasive surgery, high medical costs and without the dependence on doctors.

How Rifing works

As already mentioned, the three main fields of applications of the frequencies generated by a modern Rife Machine are primarily concerned with the following:
- **Killing** or the ability to devitalize pathogens. One must think of this modality, not only whenever the pathogen is known, but also when we know or suspect that such microorganisms can be involved in the problem presented;
- **Healing** which allows you to successfully treat a huge number of physical and mental health problems that certainly cannot be linked to the presence of pathogens;
- **Detoxing** which includes all the frequencies that can help to detox from various kinds of toxins.

The current Rife Machines devices are able to generate frequencies that, thanks to powerful software, have functions that allow for many types of configurations and databases that contain thousands of frequency programs, which can be applied in different ways, and allows you to energetically rebalance an organism and bring it back into a state of well-being.

But, what is the meaning of *energy rebalancing*?
Energy has always been associated with the creation of matter and the vital force that pervades the whole universe. Any element of the inorganic and organic matter, starting from a single atom, is characterized by its own energy and therefore by specific frequencies. Consequently, every cell, every organ, has and emits its particular frequencies. The human body, in its entirety, can be considered as a complex system of vibrations created by the interference of the many, but ordered, single frequencies that compose it.

Frequencies that are not in resonance with our natural vibrations create an imbalance, a disharmony that with time becomes chronic and **becomes a disease**.
A traumatizing event or in general, a health problem, causes the effect of a distortion of the electromagnetic field that regulates chemical and genetic cellular reactions. With a Rife Machine, you can apply the correct frequencies to eliminate the distortions that produced them and restore the initial state of balance, well-being and harmony. That is why we talk about *energy rebalancing*. Working on this principle, a Rife Machine can be able to give exceptional results and, in the opinion of many users, surprising results.

Healing

In *Comparison of asymmetrical and symmetrical pulse waveforms in electromagnetic stimulation (J Orthop Res 1992; 10: 247 - 555)* it is said that pulsed electromagnetic field stimulation (PEMF) is a non-invasive therapeutic modality that has been used successfully to stimulate healing of failed unions of surgically resistant bone fractures in humans.

The objectives of this study were:
- To determine if stimulation with an impulsive asymmetric waveform was necessary for effectiveness, and
- Determine whether symmetrical stimuli can also produce a beneficial therapeutic response.

To answer these questions and to identify which asymmetric PEMF components used in the clinic produce a therapeutic response, a fibular rabbit osteotomy model was used.

The results indicated that <u>asymmetry is not necessary</u> and that even a square wave signal with reduced pulse width can stimulate increases in rigidity. The data also indicate that the main component of the signal pulse responsible for the clinical therapeutic effect is the high-amplitude, narrow-asymmetrical pulse portion of the PEMF (<u>while the orientation of the field, does not matter</u>).

This statement identified in the scientific article cited above, is particularly interesting: *"Enhancement of fracture stiffness by electromagnetic stimuli having particular amplitude and pulse widths, support the hypothesis that this specific stimulus pulses <u>convey **information**, not just energy</u> to the tissue to produce specific response(s)."*

Let us try to make a recapitulation of the essential points of this research:
- A square waveform was used, which worked very well,
- With a narrow width of the pulse;
- In addition, impulses at a certain frequency, provide *information* to tissues and cells.

These results obtainable with PEMF combine in an incredible way with those of Rifing. But while with Magnetotherapy and Pulsed Waves, there are a series of studies and research that satisfactorily give an explanation to the electrical and biological processes that lead to the empirically found therapeutic effects, very little is known about Rifing.

The technique used for killing has been well illustrated by Dr. Royal Rife, but as regards the methods and frequencies used in therapeutic healing treatments, there is little known until now, on the origins and how they act in an organism.

We will analyze certain things of Rifing in this field of application:

\# most healing programs are made up of a series of frequencies (up to 10); only in rare cases the programs are formed by a single frequency;

\# the waveform normally used by the equipment, is the square one (complete with positive and negative half-wave, or symmetrical);

\# the effects and the results obtainable with the various therapies that use electromagnetic waves, are also obtained with Rifing, but using different application methods and electrical parameters.

So there is "something" fundamentally, common to all the dozens of applications analyzed in the previous chapters, which leads to the answers, effects and identical results, that is the restoration of a condition of health, well-being and elimination of pain, which can lead to complete healing (even if this condition occurs only in a limited number of cases and in special conditions).

Information = energy

There is a simple way, which is used to explain the principle of operation of healing frequencies, through entrainment. The explanation is as follows: If two pendulum clocks are mounted on the same wall, after a certain period of time their movements will synchronize with the same oscillation frequency.

The same thing happens with two or more metronome on the same plane or with any other device with mechanical oscillations, when they are placed on a non-rigid support. Therefore, the frequencies of the two pendulums synchronize, because one carries the other.

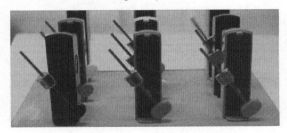

Similarly, an electromagnetic frequency known for its therapeutic properties can be used, to drag an organ, a tissue, cells, etc., to their exact "equilibrium frequency," when their energetic properties are disturbed by factors of various nature (traumas, injuries, pathologies and toxins).

If with such an explanation it is possible in a simple and immediate way to provide an explanation easily understandable to all, then this argument cannot be considered sufficient, from the scientific point of view.

All the explanations given in the previous paragraphs contribute significantly to this need for clarity, but that also the information is not yet sufficient or complete. What probably is still missing is precisely the importance of the *information* that the electromagnetic frequencies are able to give.

At this point we could venture into explanations that somehow can be provided by quantum physics, but to do so without going into too much complicated details, we will use homeopathy as a model.

Probably most of you know how a homeopathic remedy is prepared. Perhaps the principles through which these remedies act are less known. Let us make a brief summary.

To prepare a homeopathic remedy, you always start from small quantities of a substance of organic or inorganic origin and dilute it in small quantities of water. Then one drop of the first dilution is taken and further diluted with another well-defined amount of water. The procedure can continue for dozens of times, but the fundamental thing is that after each dilution, the contents of the tube is stirred or beaten (called succussion). From a physical point of view, the succussions have the function of transferring *information* from the substance of origin, to water, which has the fantastic property of recording and storing such data for a very long time (even years). Current research teaches us that these properties are obtained, thanks to the fact that water molecules are organized in clusters or in particular aggregations, able to conserve such information energetically.

We know that when the homeopathic remedy is taken, the data is then transmitted to our body, which decodes them and, if they resonate with cells or microorganisms, they cause certain curative effects, otherwise the answer will be null. It is useful to remember that apart from the in vitro experiments, homeopathic remedies work perfectly even on subjects who are not aware of what they are taking (e.g., children, the elderly or animals) and therefore the results cannot be "liquidated" as a placebo effect.

Single homeopathic remedy, based on the starting substance and dilution, can successfully treat a huge number of health problems, which will work even simultaneously on biological, pathogens and mental aspects.

But, what does this "*information*" consist of?

It is simply energy, and energy translates into frequencies, which in the case of a homeopathic remedy, these frequencies must be so many, in order to then practically act simultaneously on different aspects of human health.

Naturally, the same happens for the homotoxicology and the floral essences, but also for the essential oils and for the food we ingest; in the latter case we must always take into account that we not only have the intake of chemical substances indispensable for survival, but also a transfer, often fundamental, of energies (positive or negative).

Therefore, we have come to the conclusion that the *energies*, or the *frequencies*, are able to **inform** an organism, to modify its functions. The reason why it could be explained in a simple way is that with the fact that every atom, molecule, cell and so on, has its own energy, which can be influenced by an external field. However, regardless of the explanations that classical or quantum physics is able to offer us, the empirical results, those obtainable on the field, are certainly an undeniable scientific truth.

The experiences and successes that can be achieved with Rifing using the right frequencies and a square waveform, are practically the same as those normally obtained with Electrotherapy or Magnetotherapy, even with the latter two, very often some different electrical parameters are used (e.g., only positive half-waves, more or less long pulses, pause times, different amplitudes or field strengths, etc.).

Therefore, at least *one factor common* to all these therapies must be identified, which can then explain the reason for these identical results.

From the data resulting from the scientific publications and related experiments, it can be noted that different electrical parameters can influence the success of a treatment with electromagnetic waves. The most important of them is the waveform. In particular, <u>square and impulsive waveforms,</u> which are most often used in both Electrotherapy and Magnetotherapy.

The reason for the success of these wave types consists mainly in the rise time, which is the transition time from a low to a high level. In practice, looking for e.g., the square waveform shown above, in theory the 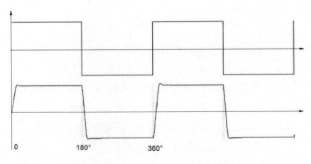 signal passes from negative to positive in a time equal to 0, so this passage is represented by a vertical line (upper image). In reality, when an electric signal makes this passage, it takes a time that cannot be equal to 0, but, for example, a few microseconds; consequently, the real transition from negative to positive will be a slightly oblique line (lower image). The steeper the "rise time" (or fall time), the more effective the waveform will be. Among all the electrical parameters that distinguish a waveform, this is the most important requirement for successful therapy.

For the same reason, different therapies such as Electrotherapy, Magnetotherapy and Rifing, can lead in many cases to identical results.

Conclusions

All the parameters that distinguish an electromagnetic wave have a series of effects on organic tissues that can be decisive for the restoration of the state of health.
These effects affect on:
- **Electrical properties** of tissues (membrane potential, ion channel opening, ion formation and displacement, injury current, etc.),
- **Biological properties** (increase in ATP, oxygenation, blood circulation, hormonal processes, etc.),
- **Gene stimulation** (repair or regeneration of cells and tissues),

However, they can also be determined by a series of **information capable of energetically modifying** cells whose electromagnetic field has been distorted by the onset of pathology.

Regarding this fundamental transfer of information, homeopathy and the practice in the applications of electromagnetic waves, teach us that an infinitesimal energy is sufficient to be implemented; a particular application of Rifing (remote transmission), addressed later, will confirm this hypothesis.
In conclusion:

The Healing frequencies used in the Rifing are able to restore a state of health or well-being thanks to all the electrical, chemical, biological and genetic principles and effects that an electromagnetic field is able to carry on living tissue
and
*to a series of **energy information** transmitted, thanks to the frequencies used.*
This last condition, by itself, is sufficient to reach the goal.

Detox

Exposure to toxins we continuously take on leads to the production of free radicals. Unless adequate amounts of cellular and extracellular antioxidants are available, free radicals begin to damage cell structures such as membranes, mitochondria, nucleic acids of DNA and cell proteins. Recent research has shown that the application of techniques using electromagnetic waves such as electrical stimulation to micro currents (MET), low-power Lasers, LEDs and infrared[44] lamps and infrasonic devices, can provide electrons with antioxidant effect.

Electromagnetic fields can strongly influence the permeability of the cell membrane, which in turn can affect the entry of nutrients and release of toxins from the cells to the extracellular matrix.

The frequency programs available with Rife Machines are used both to "move" the toxins so that they leave the occupied position (and are put back into circulation and subsequently expelled through the excretory organs), and to improve or enhance the function of organs and basic systems such as liver, kidney, intestine and lymphatic system.

In addition, some Rife Machines also feature infrared laser LEDs, with which it is possible to modulate the light at the detox frequencies, to combine the effects.

---

[44] *This photonic antioxidant effect provides an explanation of how infrared and visible light rays can be involved in the healing of various diseases.*

Killing

Dr. Royal Rife, thanks to his intuitions, his genius and his long research, has given us the resonance frequencies of dozens of pathogens, an infallible method for their devitalization and indicated the way to continue the research. Thanks to these indications, today it is possible to have thousands of programs of frequencies suitable for the killing of the same number of pathogens, while the researches are constantly evolving.

Viruses, bacteria and fungi are involved in almost all physical and mental illnesses. Regardless of whether they are the cause of a disease or if they have arrived because of the condition of a sick person, if identified and eliminated, it is possible to solve a large number of problems and in many cases create the conditions for a definitive solution of a disease.

Often the most complicated thing is to understand what the pathogen may be, which is probably the cause of the pathology found.

An example

How many people, especially when they are over fifty, suffer from backache or sciatica? The answer is obvious. Anyone who makes use of any of the techniques described in this book (From Cromopuncture to Rifing) knows very well that few applications are usually sufficient to derive great benefits that, at least for a few months, make us forget about the problem.

However, these techniques, which practically "work" on inflammation, pain or disk herniation, do not always work. Why?

One of the possible reasons is the involvement of pathogens, even in this type of pathology.

At the University Hospital of Birmingham in England, Dr. Tom Elliott, a professor of microbiology at the Birmingham hospital, found that sciatica could be caused by a bacterium, Propionibacterium acnes (the same responsible for acne). The microbiologist reports: "It is the first time that we were talking about back pain that can be caused by an infection, but remember how many surgeries we have had in the stomach, before realizing that the cause of the ulcer was a bacterium, the Helicobacter pylori, that can be defeated with antibiotics."

These bacteria normally live in hair follicles, acne or gums and can pass into the bloodstream if a person is simply brushing their teeth. They usually do not pose a threat as friendly bacteria, but when a person has a herniated disc, you start a genesis of new blood vessels that develop in the nucleus pulposus to repair the tissue. This allows bacteria to reach a disk where they can thrive, causing inflammation. They also release propionic acid, which can irritate the nerves and thus cause sciatica.

Another possible explanation for back pain comes from visceral therapy. The psoas[45] muscles, which support the column, are contiguous to the walls of the colon. This organ is the most frequent site of inflammation due to incorrect diets. Pathogens can migrate from the intestine through blood and lymph and fixate in one of the psoas muscles (left or right) causing chronic inflammation: the result is low back pain.

Infections can remain latent for months and even years and can be fixed in any tissue, including the connective and ligamentous. They can migrate from one tissue to another and remain in a subclinical state for decades, giving a blurred picture of symptoms, but yet chronic.

Based on these explanations, the principle that <u>bacteria are fixed in the inflamed areas</u> is affirmed. <u>Therefore, *they are not the cause of the problem*, but they find fertile ground in which to replicate</u> and as often happens, do not stop where everything flows, but where there is stagnation.

The strategies to be adopted

The example just described makes us understand that when utilizing therapies that use electromagnetic fields, you cannot solve a problem such as back pain or sciatica; a possible solution is the devitalization of pathogens that may be involved in this pathology.

The frequency programs available today in most Rife Machines allow you to hit a very large number of pathogens.

So, what are the best methods to deal with the killing of pathogens? The problems are of different natures.

1) The first suggestion could be to **never give up**. If we go back again to the example above: we are used to reading and hearing everything, except for an infectious nature of that type of pathology.

---

[45] *It is an internal muscle of the hip that plays the fundamental function of connecting the legs to the vertebral column.*

Beyond Rifing, *in general* this case teaches us that when:
- We perform various kinds of analyzes and nothing significant or conclusive emerges,
- With classical or alternative methods used, you cannot solve the problem,
- With Rifing frequencies, if there is not a program able to bring us back to a state of well-being, <u>then we must understand that we have taken the wrong path</u>. It is necessary to investigate deeply, to document and to consult specialists in sectors that apparently have nothing to do with the existing pathology. Psychosomatics, psychoneuroedocrinoimmunology (or PNEI) and the five biological laws, teach us, for example, that the mind and emotions can play a fundamental role in many diseases, even serious ones. So why not consult an expert in these areas or a psychologist?

In particular, one of the possibilities is to think of a cause of an infectious nature, even when nothing makes us imagine that it is possible.

2) At this point, the problem is to identify <u>what the pathogen</u> may be and how it is involved in the problem that afflicts us.

There are only two solutions: performing clinical analyzes, but when it is not possible, as in the case of viruses, finding the specialists or the means to document (in this case, even specific books or the internet, they can help us).

3) With Rifing, the application of killing frequencies involves other obstacles to overcome.

- The first concerns, <u>which frequency programs to use</u>, when our database makes available several. Regardless of the method of choice (examined later), the simplest way could be to use two or three programs at a time, to be used with the various application methods, for at least 7 days; once this cycle has been completed, one passes to the next one with three other frequency programs, until it is exhausted.

- The second occurs when the pathogens indicated as a possible cause are different. Also, in this case, as in the previous one, there is no other choice but to proceed patiently to the application of all the programs that could be useful.

At the end of this phase, all that remains is to identify the way, in which to have a confirmation of the effectiveness or not, of the treatments performed. The most immediate result (which everyone hopes for) is to see that you have eliminated the problem. When this does not happen or cannot be verified for various reasons, all that remains are to rely on clinical analyzes.

- Another question that requires attention is the choice of the various electrical parameters to be set, when possible, to obtain the best possible results.

Dr. Rife taught us that when a pathogen is hit by resonance frequencies, it vibrates to "explode" or otherwise crumble. However, these microorganisms do not remain inert when threatened by such danger. They can adapt and change, but even by slightly changing their resonance frequency, they can hide in various ways and protect themselves effectively (e.g., biofilms[46]).

This is why every Rife Machine manufacturer adopts certain strategies. The most common and effective are:

- The use of waveforms with very steep "rise time," such as the square wave or the reverse sawtooth (these waves also have the advantage of producing a very high number of harmonics, which effectively contributes to devitalization);

- The use of the eleventh harmonic: Dr. Anthony Holland has shown that when the 11th harmonic of any frequency is applied simultaneously, the "killing" results improve;

- A very limited variations of the applied frequencies (e.g., of +/- 0.02%) so that any variations in the resonance frequency of the pathogen can be included in this range. It should also be considered that the Tolerance of MOR (the Mortal Oscillatory Rate discovered by Dr. Royal Rife) within which devitalization is obtained, corresponds to a percentage of +/- 0.25% of the characteristic frequency of a pathogen. Thus by summing the two percentages, a substantially wider range is achieved within which the true coordinating resonance frequency of the pathogen is more likely to be included.

- Small sweeps, which include a very narrow range (e.g., from 99.9 kHz to 100.1 kHz) within which the resonance frequency of the pathogen is likely to be included. It is a method proposed by different authors, alternative to that of fixed frequency. Naturally, to be effective, any increase in frequency, to start from the initial one, must be lower than the percentage of MOR (0.25%) and remain on this frequency for at least 3 min (minimum time

---

[46] *A biofilm is a complex aggregation of microorganisms characterized by the secretion of an adhesive and protective matrix.*

established by Rife, so that the devitalization of a pathogen can occur), before moving on to the next one.

Finally, it is noted that there are some websites[47] that, following studies and / or measures with particular devices, have identified the resonant frequencies of various pathogens. These frequencies can then be purchased for use with its own generator.

Let us take a closer look at the last two strategies described, with an example.

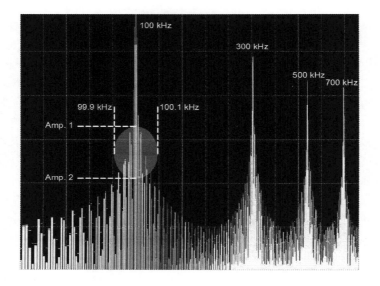

The image above represents a spectrum analysis of a square wave (details of a spectral analysis will be explained later).
The vertical white lines represent the frequencies supplied by the Rife Machine. The height of these lines is proportional to the intensity or amplitude of the signal.
The gray ellipse represents an area in which a colony of bacteria is present.
To be able to devitalize this colony, it is first necessary that:
1) The power supplied by the generator is higher than that required for the devitalization, so is superior both to that Amp1 and Amp2 (in the image this condition is satisfied);
2) The frequency is correct and is cantered with respect to the frequency range covered by the colony (in the image this condition is satisfied).

---

[47] *Two of these websites are "DNA Pathogen Frequencies" and "Frequency Foundation."*

Of course, this is <u>in many cases not enough</u> (it depends on the width of the frequency range of the bacteria colony or, in other words, on the width of the ellipse).

Observing the image and the frequency range of the colony (from 99.9 kHz to 100.1 kHz), generating a fixed frequency of 100 kHz will not be devitalized all the bacteria in the colony, so the situation could improve, but it would not be decisive. Moreover, as soon as the frequency was interrupted, the situation would reoccur as before.

At this point it is clear that a sufficient frequency oscillation or, better, a small sweep, for example from 99.7 kHz to 100.3 kHz, could guarantee the devitalization of the entire colony of bacteria.

As we will see further below, we have no certainty that the frequencies identified by Dr. Rife or those proposed by the frequency databases are the fundamental ones of devitalization. Most likely, in fact, they are sub-harmonics, or submultiples of the real frequency of killing. The question may not be a problem, because the higher harmonics of the fundamental frequency delivered by the generator could do with this task, but naturally it is essential that such harmonics have sufficient intensity for this purpose.

Considering this example and observing this image, it could be that we know that the devitalization frequency is 100 kHz, but that the real devitalization frequency is 700 kHz. In this case, if a square wave is used, which then produces a harmonic of 700 kHz, the bacteria would be devitalized only if the amplitude of this harmonic is higher, as already mentioned, is both at Amp1 and at Amp2 (naturally in this hypothesis, we must imagine the gray ellipse moved at the frequency of 700 kHz).

Bob Haining of the British Rife Research Group, at the end of 2016 published a document that reveals the discovery that the most accurate frequency for the BX virus is 12.832 MHz. Bob subsequently published the success of using this frequency with a harmonic of a carrier wave.
Therefore, the true fundamental frequency of the BX virus could be higher than 4 octaves compared to the known one of 1,604 MHz.

One thing is certain:

<u>*Even a harmonic of a frequency, if of sufficient intensity, can devitalize a pathogen.*</u>

Therefore, it might not matter if the one we are using is a fundamental frequency or a harmonic. However, we need to know that if, for example, we think that the frequency of 1 MHz is that of devitalization, but in reality the real resonance of the pathogen is 8 MHz, i.e., the octave higher harmonic (or third octave higher), then our generator must be powerful enough to perform the task.

In fact, every harmonic produced by a fundamental, loses power as it becomes higher, so to devitalize a pathogen, it must have a higher intensity than would be sufficient, if the real killing frequency was applied directly.

Let us try to make some other considerations. The bacteria reign includes unicellular microorganisms, usually of the order of a few micrometres, which can range from about **0.2 µm** of mycoplasmas up to **30 µm** of some spirochetes. A frequency that has a wavelength of 10 µm corresponds to about 30,000 GHz (we are in the infrared range). However, is there any relationship between the size of an object and its resonance frequency? I assume yes, but I have no knowledge of it (I recall the very high frequencies of the Biophotons, identified by Prof. Popp). However, if that were the case, then it could be assumed that the actual resonant frequencies of pathogens are much higher and, consequently, only higher harmonics of the killing frequencies used in Rifing are the true frequencies.

No problem, just hypothesize it, to try to study how to get the best results.

- If you use an application mode with electrodes (or something similar), you have the advantage of being able to use a square wave, which by its nature has a very high emission of higher harmonics, which therefore "naturally" approaches the emitted frequency to the real resonance of the pathogen. Since with this mode, there are no power problems (a small signal emission is sufficient), and the only limit is the maximum frequency that the generator can supply: the higher the frequency range, the better the killing capacity will be.

- With the plasma tube, the sine wave is usable, while the limit is represented by the maximum frequency of emission of the same; in this case, the limitations could be higher than in the previous case. To make up for these limitations, we need an adequate power source since, as already mentioned, *a harmonic must have sufficient intensity, to devitalize a pathogen.*

Never give up

We conclude this topic in the same way it started. For this reason it is good to know that there are also methods that allow us to perform a personalized analysis of the pathogens present in the organism and to identify the frequencies. In addition to Non-Linear Systems (NLS), already examined, some Rife Machines have Biofeedback systems able to do this type of analysis. In principle they are based on responses of our organism to electrical signals with sine wave, sent via metal or adhesive electrodes (TENS).

A machine[48] that I have had the opportunity to verify its effectiveness was based on the principles of Bioimpedanceometry, which I previously carefully examined. Unlike the device that uses a fixed frequency for its analysis, it is intended for the Biofeedback of this Rife Machine to use a scan ranging from a few kHz to some MHz. In this way, when the impedance of the organism or of the analyzed tissue is "disturbed" or "modified" by the presence of pathogens, the machine memorizes that frequency and then repurposes it, thanks to software. Each frequency identified corresponds to the precise resonance frequency of a pathogen. Of course, it is not currently possible to know the type of each pathogen identified and therefore whether it is harmful or not. In any case, the application of those memorized frequencies will result in their devitalization. This simple but ingenious process can allow you to solve another large number of infections (especially if localized).

Final considerations:

Although the modern Rife Machines are built with advanced technologies and therefore with a precision and reliability certainly higher than that available almost a century ago, I do not believe that, the results obtained by Dr. Rife are comparable to those that can be obtained today.

In this regard, reading any testimony on the subject, while noting that a modern Rife Machine can solve a huge number of health problems, I realized that the more serious the problem, the lower the chances of success.

Some hypothesize that Rife's successes were not based on frequency accuracy but on accuracy in hitting the target and natural frequency mutations. For these reasons I am convinced that the current technology still has to progress or, worse, I suspect that we are not aware of all the notions that Dr. Rife possessed (this does not

---

[48] *This is the new "GX" frequency generator of the Rife devices,* **Spooky2**.

exclude that there are people who know the original application methods).

I am equally convinced that we are very close to the discovery of the details that we still lack and the effort of many independent researchers, who will soon be able to offer us the right key.

The Herxheimer reaction

From the name of the German physician Karl Herxheimer, the Herxheimer reaction (or Herx) can basically be considered a side effect of an antibiotic treatment - be it pharmaceuticals, herbal products, colloidal silver or long exposures to the Rife technology, with killing frequencies.

When these treatments kill microbes in your body faster than the drainage system is able to remove them, these manifestations usually produce flu-like symptoms. These effects may include headache, joint pain / swelling, swollen glands, constipation, fatigue, drowsiness and many other discomforts.

Many people who are in good physical / systemic condition may not have any noticeable Herx effects.

Those who do not enjoy excellent health (even if they do not realize it) can suffer with some discomfort. Relief usually occurs within a few hours of discontinuation of therapy / treatment; in this case, drinking large quantities of water helps the system to eliminate toxins more easily.

It is desirable for the patient to resume treatment, but with a smaller dose or exposure, alternating with long pauses.

However, many of those who have experienced long chronic diseases, see these side effects as an _indicator that what they are doing is working_ and try to maintain a tolerable level of discomfort until they have a remission of their condition.

The people who have suffered for so long with Candida are more likely to witness this effect of the "death" of a large number of micro-organisms. This happens because Candida is very often dominant and therefore has all the time to devastate the immune system and the digestive tract, reducing the body's ability to manage their death.

When using Rife technology, the first rule is to proceed slowly. Using a few frequencies for a total of 10 to 15 minutes per treatment is a wise thing. Wait a day to see what it feels like. If you do not experience any of the above symptoms, the next day you can perform another session by adding more frequencies. If you have a Herx effect, wait until it has passed before continuing the treatments.

Just remember that if you initially feel worse, it means that the Rife Machine is working. It is the result of the cleaning of all the unwanted "guests."

When Rife Machines kill germs, cells often increase their permeability; this allows the expulsion of any poisons or toxins contained in the body. The application of frequencies for detoxification often has a similar result. We all have toxic substances, which have accumulated in our body year after year. The frequencies of

Detoxing are designed to release these toxins into the blood for subsequent removal. Our body has several natural mechanisms to remove these poisons, but eliminating all toxic substances takes time. During this period, symptoms present in the body, such as flu-like sensation, heavy perspiration and night sweats, fever, with or without chills, headache, malaise, diarrhea, nausea and vomiting, joint and bone pain, itching, flushing, heat and redness of the skin. Usually these symptoms will only happen at the beginning of a new treatment. The reactions will soon tend to stop and then you will feel better within a few days.

Not everyone feels this reaction. This means that there is not a large population of microorganisms, and the programs selected are the right ones. The excretory organs will work well to eliminate toxins quickly and efficiently.

The following recommendations may help during a treatment:
1. Be sure to perform a detox program before and/or during treatment.
2. Increase the break time or reduce the duration of treatments, if necessary. It is useless and harmful to put a strain on the body's capacity.
3. Drink a lot of distilled water or water and lemon.
4. Eat natural foods that can help maintain the biodiversity of the intestinal flora and eliminate toxins. Foods rich in fibers help the function of the excretory system.

The frequencies of Rifing

We have seen that the first and fundamental element of *information* transmitted to our cells, by electromagnetic waves is **frequency**.
In Rifing, it is rare for a program to consist of one or a few frequencies. Normally the programs to be applied to try to solve a specific health problem are composed of about 10 frequencies.

If you perform a search on the web, it is very easy to identify and consult different databases with long lists of names of diseases, organs, systems, etc., followed by the corresponding frequencies to be applied to try to solve them. In my book "*The frequencies of Rifing*," published in 2016, I tried to collect all the data that I was able to identify and after a long and complicated cataloging, I managed to list almost 7000 entries.

How were these frequencies identified? Why are there so many frequencies for each pathology? What is the purpose of using so many? Can they be harmful?

All those who approach this technology pose these same questions. Me too, but I have never been able to find explanations that have fully satisfied me, perhaps simply because I have never had the pleasure of meeting one of the authors of these programs.

After some years of study, I arrived at the conclusions or deductions that I will illustrate below, which is to be considered therefore only as personal opinion and not as absolute truth.

§ *How were these frequencies identified?*
The modalities with which the frequencies of healing, detoxing and killing have been obtained are the most disparate.
- Regarding healing and certainly detoxing, I have often found a perfect match between frequencies mentioned in scientific publications and those used in Rifing programs. Therefore, one of the main sources of these frequencies is certainly that of the international scientific world. It is well known that from the early twentieth century to today (thanks to scientists like Rife and Lakhovsky), the experiments and researches carried out with electromagnetic waves and with the various application methods, are in the thousands. This precious information should not be forgotten, so they were wisely collected by the various authors who created the Rifing programs.
- Another part certainly comes from research carried out in countries such as Russia,

where it is not easy to obtain scientific publications. Then there are frequencies discovered by public or private research laboratories for the most different purposes, which however have been tested for its effectiveness, before the diffusion.

- Even for killing frequencies, identifying the sources is not easy. Apart from the few tens of frequencies discovered by Dr. Rife and Dr. Hulda Clark, all the others have been identified by the most diverse means, such as electronic devices (also of a quantum type), Bioresonance devices, etc.

In any case, regardless of the origins of all the frequencies used in the Rifing, what is important is that most of them have been tested before diffusion and the proof is given simply by the effectiveness and the results they produce.

§ Why are there so many frequencies for each pathology?

The reason why each program contains (in most cases) a high number of frequencies is probably that in this way we try to implement all the possibilities available to solve a problem. According to this criterion, a Healing program can have some frequencies that directly affect the problem, others (of aid) that can be used to activate or improve the functioning of organs, tissues, cells or systems (e.g., improvement of blood circulation or system immunity, drainage of toxins, oxygenation, etc.), others that are intended to target any pathogens that may be present or otherwise involved in a problem that apparently has nothing to do with viruses, bacteria or fungi.

Similarly, the same principles are used for killing.

Furthermore, support frequencies have been added in many programs (727/728, 784/786/787, 880, 464/465) indicated for the devitalization of common pathogens, of which it is very likely to be infected. Of course, it comes to harmonics, which often also have undergone rounding.

Other programs, to end a session, use cleansing, relaxation and general well-being frequencies such as 304, 5000, 10000 and 3176.

§ What is the purpose of using so many?

At this point, the purpose appears clear. A Rifing program is normally composed of different frequencies, because this greatly increases the probability of obtaining success from the proposed treatment. Of course, sometimes this is not enough: the appropriate choice of several other factors will be those that can further increase the percentage of successes obtainable.

§ *Can they be harmful?*

The fear that the frequencies applicable with the Rifing may in some cases cause damage, is certainly legitimate, given what you hear about mobile phones, radio links, Wi-Fi, etc. Considering what is stated in the paragraph on "Harmful effects," it can be said that no cases of such effects are known in any of the applications concerning exposure to electromagnetic waves for therapeutic use (excluding contraindications). Moreover, if we reflect on the fact that each frequency is normally applied for about three minutes (even if sometimes repeated cyclically) it is understood that under these conditions, absolutely no damage can be created. In the worst case, there is no result, since the energy of the signal sent, not finding its resonance frequency, will simply be lost.

The only side effect that you could have using Killing frequencies, would be the Herxheimer effect. Should this effect occur, it is sufficient to interrupt the treatment until the physical conditions have improved.

Waveforms

When a frequency program is to be run, a series of doubts may arise about the best waveforms to be used in the various cases of healing, killing and detoxing.

Each waveform has a different function: the following indications can be useful to make the right choice.

Let us start with **Killing**.

A **square wave** is obtained by adding to a sinusoidal (fundamental) wave, the odd harmonics, and in particular the third with amplitude equal to one third of the fundamental, 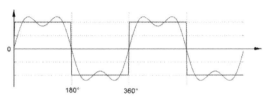 the fifth harmonic with amplitude equal to one fifth, and so on (amplitude inversely proportional to the frequency). So, a square wave is characterized by a very large number of odd harmonics.

A **sawtooth** wave, on the other hand, contains a very large number of harmonics, both odd and even, of the fundamental frequency and the amplitude of these harmonics does not decrease as rapidly as for the square wave.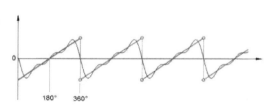

With the characteristics described above, it can be understood that both waveforms lend themselves very well to killing, given that having a very high number of harmonics means repeatedly striking the pathogen and reaching very high frequencies, that is, approaching that which is probably the real frequency of Coordination Resonance (MOR) typical of the microorganism.

To better understand what has been affirmed so far, it is important to observe, with an analysis of the electromagnetic spectrum, which are the real frequencies generated by these waves and, above all, the *intensity* or amplitude of the harmonics, which are generated.

The following images depict a spectrum analysis of the frequencies generated by different waveforms. On the horizontal axis the scale of frequencies in the range from 0 to 22 kHz is represented, while the vertical one represents the gain in decibel (which corresponds to the intensity or amplitude of the signal).

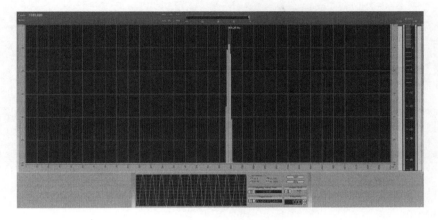

This is the spectral analysis of a **Sinusoidal** signal at a frequency of 1000 Hz. As can be seen, the image shows a single peak at 1 kHz, which is therefore the only frequency present or emitted by a generator.

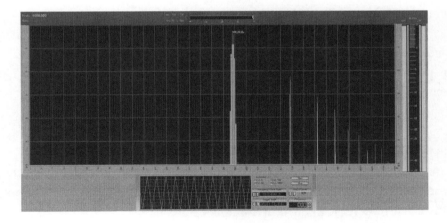

This is the spectrum of a 1 kHz **Triangular** wave. Some harmonics of decreasing amplitude are noted, at about 3 kHz, 4 kHz, 7 kHz, etc.
The amplitude of the fundamental frequency is slightly lower than that of a sine wave.

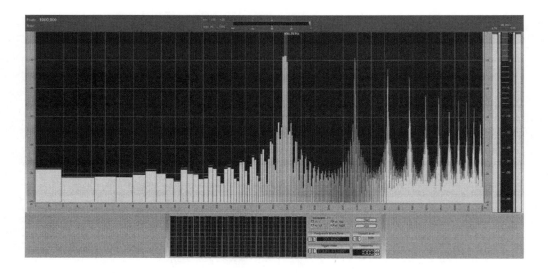

This is the spectrum of a **Square** wave, at 1 kHz. Now we can clearly see what was outlined in the theory, that is, the fundamental frequency is followed by the third harmonic (3 kHz), then the fifth (5 kHz), the seventh, etc. Of course, in the image, you can see up to the twenty-first harmonic, but if the spectrum were wider, you would see the successive odd harmonics, of ever-lower amplitude.

Another significant detail is that the fundamental frequency (1 kHz) has the maximum possible amplitude (like a sine wave).

It is also noted, by looking at the image, which, for example, the third harmonic does not have amplitude equal to one third of the fundamental (as explained above); this is not an error in the graphical representation but in the use of a decibel[49] scale. Without going into mathematical explanations, it may suffice to know that +/- 3 dB, corresponds to a doubling or halving of the power involved. So a harmonic of amplitude equal to one third of the fundamental, in a decibel scale, will have a width less than 5 dB less than the fundamental.

In conclusion, do not be fooled by the height of the harmonics represented in these images, because in reality what may seem a small difference in amplitude is actually a sharp decrease in the power emitted.

---

[49] *Logarithmic unit used to measure the relationships between the powers of two signals, sinusoidally variable over time, in particular of electric powers.*

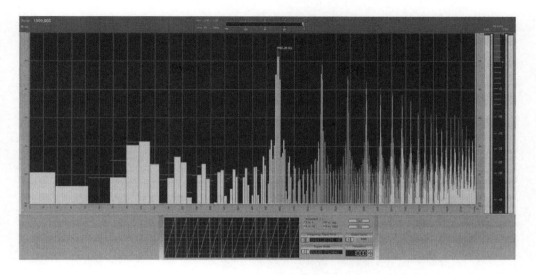

This is the spectrum of a **Sawtooth** wave, at 1 kHz. The even harmonics (2, 4, 6, 8 kHz, etc.) and the odd harmonics 3, 5, 7, 9 kHz, etc.), follow one another with a width greater than those of the square wave; so even if the fundamental does not reach the maximum, we obtain practically twice the number of harmonics (twice because both the odd and even harmonics are present).

It should also be noted that, from the spectral analysis, there is no difference between a straight and an inverted sawtooth wave.

Further reflections on the effectiveness in the killing of the Square and Sawtooth waves can arise by looking at the spectral analysis at a frequency of 6 kHz.

Square wave

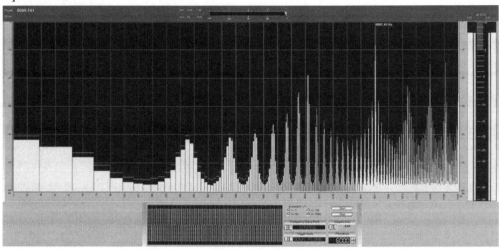

Sawtooth wave

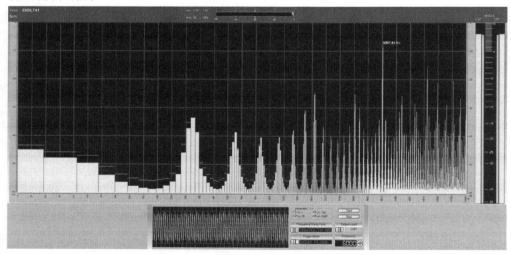

Things get complicated. Although the main harmonics of both waveforms (6 kHz x3 = 18 kHz for the Square and 6 kHz x2, 6 kHz x3 for the Sawtooth) are those with greater amplitude, a considerable number of other harmonics appear, which have not negligible amplitude. Furthermore, regardless of the amplitude, the number of harmonics seems to be the same for both waveforms.

The differences decrease and the choice becomes more difficult. All that remains is to arrive at a conclusion that considers all the situations thus far observed.

Analyzing the behavior at low and high frequencies, consider the same conditions regarding the amplitude and the harmonics, which are created; it can be said that both waveforms can perform well the function of killing. In any case, the **Sawtooth** wave always remains the best.

These considerations are certainly appropriate when we talk about relatively low frequencies compared to the entire frequency range that a generator can produce. However, what happens when we reach a few million Hz? Does it still make sense to worry about producing higher harmonics, with Square or Sawtooth waves? Are frequency generators able to create these waveforms?
We begin by trying to answer the last question.

If a generator has a frequency range of 0 - 10 MHz, it means that it is able to create a sinusoidal waveform up to a maximum of 10 MHz.

For example, if you wanted to produce a square wave of 1 MHz, you realized that the machine could reproduce this wave rather imprecisely, since to create it, you would have only the 3rd, 5th, 7th and 9th harmonic (too few to get a perfect shape).

If instead we set a 10 MHz square wave on the same generator, we will display a simple sine wave with an oscilloscope.

Moreover, when we go towards the performance limit, errors, distortions and oscillations of form and frequency begin to take place. Probably all this does not involve major problems for killing, but it is good to know that exceeding certain thresholds, talking about harmonics produced by square waves, or any other form, no longer makes much sense.

We read the technical characteristics of a frequency generator, probably without paying much attention to what they can actually give in terms of performance. The datum that probably attracts our attention most is the maximum frequency that can be reached (e.g., 10 MHz or 20 MHz), however we do not imagine that the real emission of frequencies stops before the declared one. Our limited technical knowledge also makes us think that these limits can be reached by any waveform. The reality, as can be seen from the above, is very different. In fact, the limits declared by the manufacturers of frequency generators refer exclusively to sine waves. When instead of a square or triangular wave that must be produced (now that you know that starting from a fundamental sinusoid such forms are created by the sum of a series of harmonics), you can understand that the maximum achievable frequency will be much lower than the maximum declared (unless otherwise specified).

The above analysis gives rise to a new series of doubts about the best waveforms to be used in the various cases of *healing, killing and detoxing*, so let us clarify.

Healing

I think it is appropriate to distinguish two cases.
1) It is known that our brain is able to create a series of electromagnetic waves called Delta waves (from 0.1 to 3.9 Hz), Theta (from 4 to 7.9 Hz), Alfa (from 8 to 13.9 Hz), Beta (from 14 to 30 Hz) and Gamma (from 30 to 42 Hz).
These waves can stimulate and regulate hormonal and immune activity (Delta), regulate cellular and joint activity (Theta), improve bio-chemical activity (Alpha), regulate emotional balance Betha), facilitate learning and accentuate the processes of memorization and concentration (Gamma).
Therefore, in all cases where you could deal with mental problems (e.g., depression, anxiety, insomnia, etc.) and therefore with programs that use very low frequencies, I am of the opinion that **Sinusoidal** waves are the best for this purpose.
2) Healing frequencies can be considered, all those in which pathogens are not involved and which serve to rebalance a system (e.g., endocrine, cardiocirculatory, nervous, immune system, etc.), of cells, of an organ. In all these cases, it has now been widely demonstrated that the Square wave remains the most suitable for this purpose.
Also noteworthy are the observations of some researchers who say that the square and sawtooth waves are particularly effective in regenerating functions and tissues.

Killing

Dr. Royal Rife, Dr. Hulda Clark and several other researchers have identified that the resonance frequencies of pathogens (from fungi to viruses) may include a range from around 75 kHz to some MHz.

Despite this, in many programs involving problems in which various types of bacteria are involved (e.g., sinusitis, toothache, sore throat, etc.), it is common to find very low frequencies (in the order of a few hundred Hz). They are almost always mixed *programs with frequencies of healing and killing* in which harmonics of much higher frequencies are often present; therefore if such programs succeed in their purpose, the merit is surely to be attributed to the higher harmonics that certain waves produce.

The best are undoubtedly the Square wave and the Inverse sawtooth that, as noted by the harmonic analysis, produce even and odd harmonics that can go up to the 50th.

So when we have to run such programs, surely the best thing to do is to set up an **Inverse sawtooth** wave or, alternatively or in doubt, a **Square**.

Other doubts may arise when frequencies of a particular pathogen are used, of the order of MHz or higher. Now that we know the limits of a normal generator used for a Rife Machine, you can make a couple of observations or reasoning.

- The first is the following: if a sawtooth wave is the best solution for killing, even if beyond a certain limit, this wave is transformed by the generator into sinusoidal, patience! The essential thing is that it carries out its task and in addition, we will have the advantage of using a single waveform, in any case.

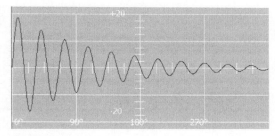

- The second is the following: if I have the certainty that the frequency I want to use is very high and I know that my generator is not able to reproduce the chosen waveform, it is better to use a **Damped Sinusoid** (the one probably used by Rife), which has the advantage of creating abrupt transitions from low to high amplitudes: this characteristic should be particularly lethal for pathogens.

Remember once again that all these arguments made on the waveforms are valid in all cases, except when a plasma tube is used (which normally emits only sinusoidal waves).

Detoxing

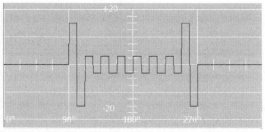

There are not many studies regarding Detoxing. Therefore, when detoxing, it is recommended to use logical reasoning and follow what is stated in the generator usage manuals, with the two preferred waveforms, which are Square and, if available, the H (also called Square H Bomb). The second is the preferred one because probably the two strong peaks that characterize it, can contribute to break the bonds that hold toxins to other molecules, within an organism.

When the frequencies do not work

The causes of non-effectiveness of a frequency program can be of various kinds. A first factor can be determined by the reliability of the PC and the software used.

The characteristics and performance of the generator follow, such as:
- The accuracy of the frequency generator: it is normal that if we set a frequency and in fact, a different one is generated, we cannot expect great results from this Rife Machine (an oscilloscope can be of great help in verifying this parameter);
- The limits in terms of performance, such as a limited frequency range, insufficient power, etc.

In addition to these technical factors, there may be a number of other causes why results cannot be achieved. The causes could be the following:

- The frequencies used are incorrect, not verified or otherwise unsuitable for the case;
- The method of application is not the most effective for this purpose;
- The settings of the electrical parameters and settings for healing or killing are incorrect;
- There are factors that do not allow the efficacy of the treatment (e.g., biofilm, in the case of pathogens);
- The **emission power** of the device used, is not sufficient to deeply reach all the infected tissues (this is an important parameter especially when using a Plasma tube).

If we think everything is correct and working, but we do not get the correct results, we simply have to think that we are very likely doing something incorrectly. An example has been described in the chapter on Killing, about the various reasons that can cause sciatica or a backache. So, before giving up, it is always good to investigate, study and consult the right professionals.

Sometimes the causes and therefore the solutions can be so simple, that we do not realize it. Vice versa when the causes are for example of genetic or mental origin, then it can be difficult to solve them, even with the Rifing.

Other cases with difficult solutions occur when a program of frequencies reduces or eliminates a symptom, but as soon as the treatments are suspended, one returns to the initial situation. It is the condition in which the true origin of the problem has not been identified and is practically equal to the classic daily intake of a drug or a supplement to mitigate a health problem. Even in this case there are not many choices. If you do not want to remain "tied" to the treatments that a machine can offer, you must try other ways, as mentioned above.

The methods of application

There are many *Rife Machines* currently on the market, which vary in price. There are systems that use only software and a sound card of a computer (so with frequencies that reach a maximum of 20 kHz) to systems that are much more complex and very expensive.

So, choosing the most efficient Rife Machine and with the best quality / price ratio, for those entering this technology, is not very simple.

Most likely, they will all work (in this sector, I do not think there are "fakes"), but what distinguishes them are the real possibilities to solve the greatest possible number of health problems. Think about it, make a simple Rife Machine, which is able to deal with a good number of situations and you will only need a few elements:
- Frequency programs are now in the public domain;
- If you do not want to be limited by the frequency range of a sound card, buy a frequency generator that will have a frequency range from 0 to some MHz, which does not represent an excessive expense;
- Finally, you will need good software that can manage databases and electromagnetic wave settings

Power, is not a factor of excessive importance since, as already mentioned, the fundamental function of these machines is to transfer *information* to cells and tissues.

It seems easy, right? Of course, with such a configuration you can only use the mode that uses the contact electrodes on the skin, to transfer electromagnetic waves; in any case, even if with many limitations, such a configuration can already give good results. According to these criteria, several simple Rife Machines are made (usually portable and battery powered).

However, once the first programs have been tested and the first successes are achieved, it is inevitable that one begins to expect more. For the purchase of a good Rife Machine, it is advisable to consider and evaluate:

- The software used and in particular: the possibility to configure all the electrical parameters of a wave, the programming of the usable sequences and above all the number of frequency programs stored in the databases;
- The characteristics of the frequency generator and in particular the maximum frequency that can be reached (at least a few tens of MHz). This parameter is very important for killing frequencies, since as mentioned above, the higher this frequency will be the possibility to generate square waves up to some MHz;
- All the devices available that can be connectable to the generator (including a plasma unit).

The devices by which frequency programs can be applied represent one of the main requirements that distinguish some evolved Rife Machines. In fact, the variety of methods of application can contribute not only to the success of the treatments performed but also to the speed with which it is possible to obtain them.

The most important accessories available are described below.

The Plasma tube

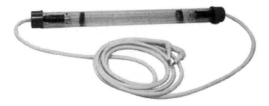

It was the first device used by Rife to devitalize pathogens. The tube acts as an antenna that combines photon emission with electromagnetic and plasma waves. By keeping the tube at a distance very close to the body and using the appropriate frequencies, it is possible to devitalize the pathogens responsible for even very serious diseases.

The apparatus capable of powering and managing this transmission device is a high voltage signal amplifier, which connects to the frequency generator. To be efficient and emit the frequencies identified by Rife or other researchers, it must be able to work up to some MHz. Among the various accessories that can be connected to a Rife Machine, it is the most powerful and effective way to eliminate fungi, viruses and bacteria.

The electrodes for contact mode

In the years when Royal Rife began the collaboration with John Crane, a method of frequency application was introduced, much simpler and cheaper than the plasma tube: the cutaneous electrodes (introduced in 1958 on a new generator built by Crane).

In this way, the electromagnetic energy is transmitted through electrodes that can be constructed of various kinds of materials: surgical steel cylinders, metal plates or adhesive skin electrodes. With this type of mode, it is possible to apply frequencies of Healing, Killing and Detoxing without any frequency limit (the limit is simply that of the generator).

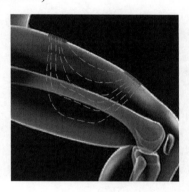

Considering that the modern Rife Machines can generate frequencies from 0 to some tens of MHz, it is understood that with such a range it is possible to include almost all types of Electrotherapy (of course in this case it is Healing applications). Moreover, if the software allows the programming of the waves and of the parameters that can be used, it is possible to experiment with new methods of application. In particular by dosing the amplitude of the voltage or, if possible the current, one can re-enter the field of stimulation with microcurrents (MET or MENS) with all the advantages, especially at the cellular level, that the type of technology involves (as described in the paragraph dedicated, among all types of electro-stimulation, the MET is the one that can solve the greatest number of health problems). In this way, by combining MET with Rifing, it is likely that unimaginable objectives can be achieved. It is worth experimenting.

Electromagnetic devices

The Electromagnetic device is a mostly unknown and unused application, but it can provide great results in Healing and Killing. By properly connecting Magnetotherapy or PEMF devices (coils of various types and shapes) to a Rife Machine, it is possible to obtain results that are very often faster than those obtainable with classical Magnetotherapy.

This topic has been the subject of studies and research that I have carried out in recent years.

As in the one described above (combination of MET and Rifing), also in this case the idea is to mix the technologies to sum up the effects. In fact, the person who uses Magnetotherapy knows that the frequencies that are normally used are very few and are always the same, whatever the point of application. Rifing uses many frequencies, which are different for each type of problem.

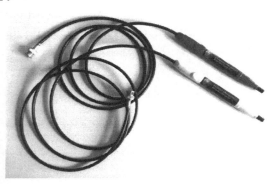

Magnetic Pen

By appropriately combining the magnetic coils with the waveforms and frequencies that Rifing makes available, you can get something different and in my opinion, more efficient than the separately used technologies. This is due to the simple fact that in this way it is possible to sum up the electrical effects in tissues, produced by a magnetic field with the ***information*** that the frequencies of Rifing are able to give.

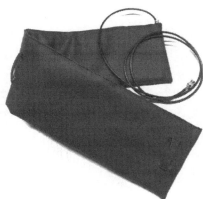

Magnetic carpet

In my latest research, I have created and designed several electromagnetic devices[50] applicable to a Rife Machine, all with exceptional results.

One in particular is proving to give very encouraging results in both Healing and Killing. It is in fact an electromagnetic mat made with completely different principles from the classical ones for use in Magnetotherapy or PEMF (made with a series of coils, arranged in the padding of the carpet). In fact, while the devices made for these applications have an emission of an exclusively magnetic field, what I have done allows an emission of an electric and magnetic field. This explains the efficiency in both Healing and Killing applications.

Other devices

Among the accessories that can be connected to a Rife Machine, there are practically no limits.
In order to improve or enhance the effects, they can in fact be connected:
- Laser LEDs with specific wavelengths, which pulsing at the frequency set by the generator, can sum up the effects of both technologies (the most frequent and effective use, above all it concerns the pathologies of the skin);
- Infrared led carpets, which at low frequencies can create effects similar to those described above;
- Ultrasonic devices, which can also emit frequencies up to 1 MHz, which are useful for the Healing and the Killing;
- Devices for imprinting magnetic bands, or water (to obtain effects similar to homeopathic products);
- Devices for the production of colloidal silver;
- Radionics devices;
- Signal amplifiers, which in certain cases or applications may be useful for accelerating the effects.

---

[50] *The main devices designed and tested are: a device for imprinting magnetic cards, a Pen, a Coil for joints and a Carpet, magnetic. Other devices and methods of application are currently under study and experimentation.*

Remote transmission

According to Ross Adey, cell membrane glycoproteins[51] act as molecular chemical receptors, but also as antennas of electromagnetic or electrical fields. In this way, the cells can function both as receivers and as transmitters.

Cell receptors can be activated by electric fields characterized by particular frequencies through a process known as electro-conformational coupling (Tsong, 1989), as if activated by a chemical signal. Furthermore, this electrical property of cell membrane receptors would allow cells to scan incoming frequencies and then fine tune their circuits to allow them to resonate at particular frequencies (Charman, 1996).

In addition to these studies, which explain how local electrical signal reception can take place, there are others that describe the possibility that such transmission may occur at a distance.

As reported by the German biophysicist Prof. **Fritz Albert Popp**, the cells of an organism, are able to emit and receive very weak radiations of light (biophotons), by means of DNA, which acts as a transceiver station, allowing constant electromagnetic communication both inter-cellular and with the outside world (even long-distance).

According to several scholars, one of which is Prof. **Georges Lakhovsky**, the double helix of DNA behaves like a dipole. This structure is able to generate and propagate electromagnetic waves in the surrounding environment. The DNA with its double-helix structure, has its own value from the chemical point of view, but certainly also from the physical point of view, generating electromagnetic waves to convey information within an organism (therefore cells exchange information in real time, not only through the nervous system, but above all through electromagnetic signals).

Hence, the DNA double helix acts as an antenna able to transmit and receive coded information of energy signals, via *non-local space*[52].
When using these principles, it is possible to use a Rife Machine to "transmit" information remotely, using a simple device (remote). The method consists in investing a biological sample that contains DNA, combined with the energy of the frequencies; then instantly this energy is transmitted, via non-local space, to the

---

[51] *Glycoproteins are created from the interaction of membrane proteins and membrane carbohydrates*

[52] *Non-local space has been defined as "dark" energy (dark because it is outside the electromagnetic spectrum and therefore cannot be observed or measured). Nikola Tesla called it "the mind of God."*

owner of that DNA.

The devices for operating in the "remote" mode are able to use the enormous potential of scalar waves to make this remote transmission even more effective. Such waves are difficult to measure with orthodox means and behave like a super-compressed signal both for the energy of the frequencies and for the transmission capacities of the DNA.

Albert Einstein called it "Spooky action at a distance." Modern physics calls it "quantum entanglement." In other words, this means that if any part of a single system is removed from that system and placed in a different position, every action performed on that part will instantly have effects on the system and vice versa.

Similarly, when the energy of the frequencies is applied to a sample with DNA, that *information* will be transmitted instantly and without spatial limitations (i.e., without limits of distance) exclusively to the subject with that DNA.

This special Remote device has been designed, tested and implemented by an international Team[53] of designers.

This means that all the frequency programs available with a Rife Machine can be applied to an organism without having any physical contact.

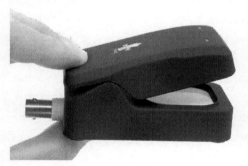

The effectiveness of such a futuristic and revolutionary device is in most cases surprising. Using the principles, which are described above, it is plausible that sometimes it is a bit slower or less effective than the other modes of application, but considering the convenience of use, a Remote device is truly unique.

In the application practice, there are both cases of extreme sensitivity and very rare cases of inefficiency, but these conditions represent less than 10% of users who have used it for years.

---

[53] *The Remote and Scalar devices have been designed by Team* ***Spooky2****, which produces one of the best known Rife Machines.*

Scalar Wave technology

The device just described, is not the only way to use Scalar Waves for treatments of any kind. Recently, the same Team[18] of researchers that had developed the Remote; had devised an apparatus capable of producing scalar waves for treatments able to give even better effective solutions, in case the health issues are of a more complex nature.

As already mentioned in the first chapter, scalar waves, besides having the ability to transfer energy, are also able to transfer *information*, since DNA is a perfect scalar antenna. Scalar energy improves the natural potential to promote healing[54]; it does so by strengthening the natural electrical charges in the cells, improving the circulation and cellular metabolism: in practice, giving an organism the energy and informational charge it needs helps it re-establish its normal biological and functional processes.

Scalar energy greatly improves the functions of the mitochondria and digestive, endocrine, nervous, circulatory, immune and lymphatic systems, offering a wide range of health benefits.

In "Scalar Energy: The Science and Wonder Behind Its Benefit" (by Dr. Romerlito C. Macalinao), in addition to the effects mentioned above, a new and fundamental aspect is examined to understand how scalar waves can bring great benefits in a very high number of diseases. In this book the author, after having exposed all the benefits that oxygenation of the blood involves, disclosed a series of studies in which he demonstrates that scalar energy oxygenates the blood, contributing to the oxygen requirements of the human body that enables the organism at the cellular level to fight off disease and infection. It is the oxygen effect that allows for all the benefits of scalar energy and that explains its healing potential. People from all over the world have testified the benefits of scalar energy and the results are as follows:

- Improves cardiovascular and circulatory health; normalizes blood pressure and removes swelling and stasis
- Boosts the immune and endocrine system
- Relieves stress; enhances focus, memory and concentration

---

[54] *Effect of Non-Hertzian Scalar Waves on the Immune System - and - Biological Interactions with Scalar Energy: Cellular Mechanisms of Action - Dr. Glen Rein, Stanford University Medical Center*
- Biological Effects of Quantum Fields and Their Role in the Natural HealingProcess - Dr. Glen Rein, Quantum Biology Lab, Miller Place, NY

- Enhances memory and cognitive function and works as an antidepressant
- Improves the parasympathetic and sympathetic nervous systems
- Reduces pain, swelling and inflammation
- Anti-aging; restores cells and prevents degenerative diseases
- Normalizes body weight; increases metabolic rate and promotes weight loss
- Improves strength, flexibility, balance and endurance, i.e., athleticism
- Protects the body from e-smog and strengthens the human biofield to facilitate health and wellness.

Our cells communicate using scalar fields[55]. When this communication is blocked, our health will often deteriorate. Scalar fields introduce energy and restore this communication and the natural means of defense against an organism.

In this book, it has been repeatedly stated that the key to restoring health is *information*. With this machine, the information is provided with the appropriate scalar waves that can be further enriched with those provided by the classic Rife frequencies or medicinal products (synthetic or natural).

The application is performed by, placing oneself between a transmitting and receiving unit, in order to be completely encapsulated by the scalar field.

This is certainly the most advanced and promising technology in the world of Rifing. This research makes constant continuous progress, so I am sure the future will offer us more and more efficient and evolved equipment.

---

[55] *DNA and cell resonance: magnetic waves enable cell communication. - Meyl K. - DNA Cell Biol. 2012 Apr; 31 (4): 422-6. doi: 10.1089/dna.2011.1415.*

Conclusions

Prof. **Georges Lakhovsky** in 1926 stated that cells, tissues and organs function as micro-radios that resonate at their resonance frequency. When the cells fall ill, they vibrate at a different frequency from the natural one and to heal them they must be subjected to the right frequency, which will bring them back to vibrate at the 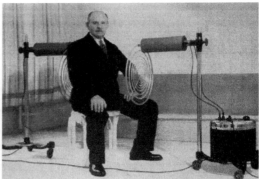 "correct" frequency. Lakhovsky designed and built an oscillator at multiple wavelengths which, by emitting innumerable harmonics, was able to resonate with any group of cells in the human body; he used it to treat many people and is still in use today.

During that same period in time, Dr. **Royal Rife** demonstrated that every elementary organic particle has its own resonance frequency and according to these principles succeeded in devitalizing pathogens that can lead to even deadly diseases.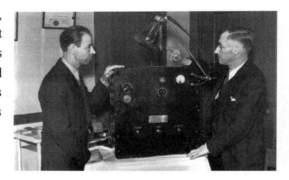

Today many contemporary scientists, like those of the past, affirm the same principle: frequencies are the key to diseases but also to healing. After so many years of darkness, science is rediscovering all this. Therapeutic machines that use electromagnetic waves to transmit their energy and / or the information they are able to provide to an organism are increasingly numerous.

Almost no one has the courage to recognize which scientists have opened the doors to these technologies; so when their imagination does not provide anything original, better call it *quantum medicine*.

Considerations on the technologies examined

After the detailed description of all the most known technologies that use electromagnetic waves, it is possible to make some observations.

- Even if what has been reported in the previous chapters tries to make a generalization of the scope of Electrotherapy and Magnetotherapy, there is almost nothing precise and definite, in the sense that every researcher or every manufacturer of such equipment gives different definitions or uses different operating principles and electrical parameters (especially waveforms, pulse duration, application times, etc.).

Therefore, by reading the scientific articles or the technical characteristics of such apparatuses, it happens that the methods used cannot be cataloged in any precise way. Naturally, this creates a bit of confusion, since often, different methods can still lead to identical results. At this point, you can ask yourself which one is the best, the fastest or the most efficient!

Unfortunately, the answer frequently does not exist simply because the only way to obtain it would be to compare methodologies and / or devices (data that are almost never available at all). In any case if, as we have seen, the mechanisms of action on cells and tissues are almost always the same; the only parameter that could give us a really important indication, would be to know the number of successes obtained and the times in which it is normally possible to reach a positive result. Here, thanks to a collection of data and information, we tried to give some answers, but we realize that the issue is not simple.

- Between Rifing and Magnetotherapy (in general) there are a series of applications that, even with different methods, principles and frequencies are able to obtain identical results that is the restoration of a state of health or well-being In the field of Magnetotherapy, the technique that distinguishes itself in a particular way compared to Rifing, is that of Pulsed Electro-Magnetic Fields (PEMF) which, thanks to a large number of scientific publications, have shown excellent abilities especially in the field of repair and regeneration of organic tissues.

In summary, if Rifing and PEMF *both succeed in successfully solving a large number of health problems* (even if in ways that are sometimes different, sometimes overlapping), the first is characterized by the excellent capacity for the *devitalization of pathogens*, while the second for the *regeneration of tissues* damaged by trauma or serious diseases. For the reasons just described these two technologies have been the most detailed.

The emission power

The power of a device that emits electromagnetic waves is a parameter that should be considered solely for the purpose and functions of the therapy.
In general, it can be said that when ***information*** is to be transferred, very low powers are sufficient to achieve the goal. On the other hand, when it is necessary to trigger bio-electric effects that must cause reactions of various kinds, then the power of electromagnetic waves and related equipment can be decisive.

Of all the applications examined so far, we see when and why it is necessary to have adequate power.
- **Therapies with light radiations**: they are all applications that require adequate power to be effective, especially those that use LEDs and Lasers. The only exceptions are Chromotherapy and Chromopuntura, where the information of the colors are used to determine the desired effects.
- **Electrotherapies**: since these electrodes are applied directly to the skin, it is normal that a very minimum mount of electrical current is sufficient, for any type of application. Indeed, in the case of microcurrent stimulation, it has been seen that if the current circulated in the affected area exceeds the threshold of just 1 mA, the effects could even be contrary.
- **Thermotherapies**: they are applications that, because they exploit the electrical characteristics of the tissues to cause their heating, need very high powers, up to over 1000W.
- **Ultrasound and Shockwave**: also in this case the power (of a few watts) must be adequate for the mechanical transfer of the vibrations produced by the equipment, to the tissues to be invested.
- **Neuroacoustics**: even if the nature of the sound waves transmitted through a headset, are predominantly informational in nature, a modest power is required for the reproduction of the acoustic pieces.
- **Magnetotherapy**: as already mentioned, they can exploit both principles with powers varying from a few picogauss to thousands of gauss.

Since a magnetic field induces in the tissues an electric field that will then serve to produce therapeutic effects, when it is intended to produce a similar effect, it is necessary that the electrical power be consistent (in this case we speak of hundreds or thousands of gauss). Power can be decisive even when it is necessary to reach deep tissues of the human body.

However, when the electrical power is intended to provide the tissues with information that is useful for gene stimulation, then fields of weak electrical intensity will be sufficient to achieve excellent results.

- **Rifing**: in Healing, the fundamental principle is to transfer energy *information* to cells and tissues, so sufficient potencies are sufficient to obtain great results. This does not exclude that having more power when using electromagnetic devices (e.g., carpets, coils, etc.), could mean combining the effects and producing faster results.

As for Killing, things are reversed only when the Plasma tube is used. In fact, acting as an antenna with its own emission waves that must reach pathogens that can be found in even deep tissues, and then destroys them (like a crystal glass invested by its resonance frequency), it is understood that adequate electrical power is needed (normally more than 40/50 W).

Biological and therapeutic effects

After examining various explanations on the biological effects and modalities of a large number of applications of electromagnetic fields, it may be useful to make a recapitulation, so it is easier to identify the best choice for every type of health problem.

Probably nobody has had a satisfactory experience in all the applications described in the previous chapters. Therefore, the following statements are just an attempt to clarify what is based on scientific research, testimonies and experiences of some therapists: for that reason, absolutely nothing is certain or definitive.

It is also specified that according to the criterion just stated, the therapeutic indications indicated below for each application are only those of greater importance, listed in order of importance (in relation to the most frequent use and / or demonstrated efficacy).

Therapies with light radiations

Biological effects:
- Production / balancing of the endocrine system - production of hormones (**Light Therapy**);
- Production of Vitamin D (**Heliotherapy**);
- Oxidative reactions only in pathological cells (**Photodynamic Therapy**);
- Activation of the mitochondrial respiratory chain and production of ATP (**LED and Laser therapy** with red / infrared light);
- Energetic activation, according to traditional Chinese medicine (**Chromopuncture, Laser therapy**).

Therapeutic indications:
- **Heliotherapy**: dermatological diseases, osteo-articular, respiratory, haematological, circulatory system and mood disorders.
- **Light Therapy**: alteration of the sleep-wake rhythm and the circadian rhythm, mood disorders and mental disorders.
- **Photodynamic therapy**: dermatological diseases, pre-tumor lesions and tumor lesions.
- **Phototherapy**: jaundice, dermatological diseases and cosmetic treatments.
- **Chromotherapy**: rebalancing of chakras and psychosomatic disorders.
- **Chromopuncture**: diseases of various kinds.
- **LED and Laser therapy**: wounds and dermatological diseases, inflammations and diseases of various kinds.

Electrostatic Therapy

Biological effects:
- Actions of an excitomotor type, vasomotor (vasodilatation) and antalgic-sedative;
- Repolarizing effect on cells;
- Increase in the arterial flow of the district;
- Anti-edema effect (which reduces water retention).

Therapeutic indications:
- Cellular metabolism and microcirculation stimulation;
- Type 2 diabetes;
- Anti-inflammatory and acceleration of hematoma absorption;
- Pathologies of various kinds.

Electrotherapies

Biological effects:
- Increase in ATP (**MET**);
- Improvement of amino acid transport through the membrane and increase of cellular protein synthesis (**MET**);
- Biological repair and recovery of damaged cells and tissues with similar effects to injury current (**MET**);
- Excitomotor action on muscle fibers (**NMES, H-wave**);
- Electrical stimulation to nerves that feed paralyzed muscles (**FES**);
- Blocking of the transmission of painful impulses and generation of endorphins (**TENS, PENS, PNT and HVGS**);
- Stimulation of the hypothalamus to the production of neuro-hormones (substantial increases in beta endorphins, adrenocorticotrophic hormone and serotonin) (**CES**).

Therapeutic indications:
- **(MET) Micro Current Electrical Stimulation**: attenuation of acute and chronic pain, reduction of inflammation, edema, lesions, bedsores, ulcers, wounds, neuropathies, arthritis and bursitis, regeneration of damaged tissues and lifting effect.
- **(NMES) Neuromuscular Electrical Stimulation Devices**: increase in muscle strength and range of motion, correction of spastic contractures, dysphagia, and neuromuscular stimulation in children with cerebral palsy.
- **(FES) Functional Electrical Stimulation**: Stroke, Multiple Sclerosis (MS), Spinal Cord Injury, Cerebral Palsy and Parkinson's disease.
- **(TENS) Transcutaneous Electrical Nerve Stimulation**: attenuation of acute and chronic pain.
- **(CES) Cranial electrotherapy stimulation**: mood disorders, mental disorders, brain injuries, fibromyalgia, multiple sclerosis (experimental), quit smoking and for opiate withdrawal.
- **H-wave**: stimulation of muscles and nerves, to promote circulation and alleviate pain, muscle sprains, temporomandibular joint dysfunction, reflex sympathetic dystrophy and diabetic ulcers.
- **(PENS) Percutaneous Electrical Nerve Stimulation**: attenuation of acute and chronic pain.
- **(PNT) Percutaneous Neuromodulation Therapy**: chronic non-treatable pain relief, as an auxiliary treatment in post-operative or post-traumatic pain management.

- **(HVGS) High Voltage Galvanic Stimulation**: treatment of acute and chronic pain and reduction of edema.
- **(EAP) Electroacupuncture**: diseases of various kinds
- **Electrostimulation of acupuncture points**: diseases of various kinds.

Thermotherapies

Biological effects:
- Increase in the temperature of even deep tissues;
- Damage or destruction of cancer cells;
- Release of cytokines which stimulate the arrival of leukocytes on the heated zone;
- Analgesic effect for reduction of conduction in sensory nerve endings;
- Acceleration of cell metabolism;
- Vasodilation;
- Deep hyperemia.

Therapeutic indications:
- **Infrared rays**: decubitus sores, arthropathies, muscular contractures, cutaneous trophic disorders and oncological therapies (with the Laser).
- **Radar therapy or Microwave**: Traumas, osteo-articular and muscular diseases and Raynaud's disease.
- **Marconitherapy**: Circulatory alterations, inflammation, infections, chronic arthrosis, trauma, Herpes Zoster and Bell's palsy.
- **Tecar-Therapy**: Traumas, osteo-articular and muscular pathologies, and from venous and lymphatic insufficiency.
- **Oncological hyperthermia**: most of the deep solid tumors, superficial solid tumors, haematological tumors, skin and bone metastases.

Ultrasound

Biological effects:
- Mechanical: micromassage and microconstructions with acceleration of metabolism and cell reproduction;
- Thermal: vasodilation, superficial and deep vascularization, pain reduction;
- Chemical: modification of pH and permeability of cell membranes.

Therapeutic indications:
- Disaggregation of calcifications (lithotrissia);
- Fibrolytic effect (dissolution of thrombus);

- Trauma, osteo-articular and muscular pathologies;
- Aesthetic applications.

ESWT - Extracorporeal Shockwave Therapy

Biological effects:
- Angiogenesis (development of new blood vessels);
- Acceleration of cell metabolism;
- Regeneration and tissue repair;
- Multiplication and differentiation of stem cells.

Therapeutic indications:
- Disaggregation of calcifications (lithotrissia) - kidney stones;
- Erectile dysfunction;
- Cellulitis and for body remodeling;
- Tendon and related diseases, even in the absence of calcifications;
- Pain, persistent edema and joint stiffness after surgery;
- Healing of chronic wounds, burns and diabetic ulcers.

Neuroacoustics

Biological effects:
- Rebalancing of organs, tissues and cells, with various stimulation effects;
- Revitalization of neuronal connections, synchronization of the hemispheres of the brain.

Therapeutic indications:
- Removal of psycho-emotional blocks;
- Increase in physical-postural balance;
- Induction of a healthy and deep sleep;
- Energy balance of the chakras and rebalancing of the aura;
- Diseases of various kinds.

Magnetotherapy

Biological effects:
- Repair and regeneration of tissues, thanks to the stimulation of gene expression; restoration of the membrane potential towards optimal values, with oxygenation and ATP;
- Activation of ion channels with ion formation and displacement;
- Vasodilation and neoangiogenic effect (reinvigorates the walls of blood

vessels);
- o Antalgic effect.

Therapeutic indications:
- Delays in the consolidation of fractures, stimulation of bone regeneration, improvement of bone density;
- Osteo-articular and muscular pathologies of any kind;
- Attenuation of acute and chronic pain;
- Localized inflammation with improvement of vasodilation, angiogenesis and blood oxygenation;
- Central and peripheral nervous system disorders with tissue regeneration / repair;
- Mood disorders, mental and psychiatric disorders;
- Dermatological diseases;
- Infections and diseases of various kinds.

Rifing

Biological effects:
- o Devitalization of pathogens (fungi, bacteria and viruses);
- o Functional rebalancing of cells and tissues;
- o All the effects of Electrotherapy and Magnetotherapy.

Therapeutic indications:
- Pathologies of infectious origin or related to the presence of pathogens;
- Pathologies of any nature;
- Detoxification of heavy metals and toxins.

Final reflections

Probably many of you, before reading this book, did not imagine that electrical currents and electromagnetic fields had such distant origins and so many modes of application. However, do not think that everything is included in this book, on the contrary those described in these pages, more or less in depth, are only the best known therapies. I frequently read about very new machines in use in hospitals, which thanks to the electromagnetic waves are able to "cure" even very serious diseases. They are almost always built in a nation that is not ours and that cost millions of euro or dollars: this is enough for them not to be branded as something whose technology is based on "nothing."

Let us not talk about apparatuses based on quantum physics theories! For many doctors, just saying these words, is cause for them to sink into a total skeptic depression.
Reading this book, I am sure that many have thought that some of the topics covered here are scientifically lacking. Yet, according to science, for an experiment to be considered "credible" it must be "repeatable" that means that other researchers in other parts of the world must be able to replicate the same experiment and achieve the same results. So experimenting, in many cases, does not cost so much! However, there are those who probably do not wish to popularize the spread of these types of treatments.
Magnetotherapy, in many countries is still considered an "experimental" technology.
For Rifing, things are even worse, because very few nations recognize their effectiveness.

There are currently millions of people or therapists in the world who successfully use all the therapies described in this book, but very often, they do so in secret, because they risk credibility, seriousness or professionalism.
I am a skeptic, because I come from a "classical" scientific training. Nevertheless, I have an open mind, so if someone proposes to me, something that I can hardly believe, I personally want to experience the effectiveness, before classifying it in any way. Only after having found what "works," then can I dedicate myself to perform all the research that can give me a scientific explanation. That is why people make me smile, when they tell me "I do not believe in homeopathy" or

"I do not believe in Rifing." What is there to believe? We are not talking about UFOs, ghosts or miracles, but of science and therefore of phenomena that can be tested and above all has been proven to be repeatable!

What is the percentage of people who benefit from a given drug? 60 or 70%? And, from these therapies? As was mentioned before, if not superior.

So there is nothing in which to believe or not, what I could suggest to those who have doubts about any of these therapies is to try them, as I did. Then you can see for yourself the real effectiveness, the success rates, the speed with which a problem can be solved and all the cases that have had poor or difficult success. One thing I have certainly seen over the years that I dedicated myself to the research and experimentation of these technologies, is that the success rate is directly proportional to the technical knowledge of the equipment used and the studies in medicine and naturopathy that you have.

Then, if the technology is valid and it leads to good results, you will almost certainly be able to establish credibility and success.

ABOUT THE AUTHOR

Marcello Allegretti, electrical engineer and naturopath, is an independent scientific researcher and owner of a bioengineering and energetic rebalancing laboratory.

Stimulated by a strong personal motivation, he devoted many years to the study of traditional medicine, alternative and complementary, but above all to technologies for the use of electromagnetic waves in the field of energy medicine, that is intended as a means for rebalancing for psycho-physical well-being. .
In the course of his research, he has designed and implemented several electromagnetic devices applicable to frequency generators, able to provide results much higher than those obtainable from similar devices.

Author of the book "The Frequencies of Rifing" published in the US in March 2016, and successfully sold all over the world.

He is one of the leading experts in Italy of the technology born from the research of Dr. Royal Rife and an Italian consultant of an international team of engineers, designers and technicians for the study, research and development of bioengineering technologies for the use of electromagnetic frequencies for human well-being.

© 2018 Ing. Marcello Allegretti

All rights reserved. No part of this book shall be reproduced, stored in a retrieval system, or transmitted, by any means, mechanical photocopying, electronic, digital scans, or otherwise without written permission of the author.

Cover design *Marco Allegretti*

Printed in Poland
by Amazon Fulfillment
Poland Sp. z o.o., Wrocław

29217454R00087